SERIES ON MEDICINE, PSYCHOLOGY AND RELIGION

MARRIAGE and the FAMILY

MEDICINE, PSYCHOLOGY, RELIGION:

New Directions, New Integrations

Edited by
John T. Chirban

HOLY CROSS ORTHODOX PRESS
Brookline, Massachusetts 02146
1983

50 Goddard Avenue
Bookline, Massachusetts 02146

Published by the Holy Cross Orthodox Press.

Library of Congress Cataloging in Publication Data
Main entry under title:

Marriage and the family; Medicine, psychology,
religion.
(Series on Medicine, psychology, and religion)
Based on the annual Symposium on Medicine, Psychology, and Religion held in 1983.
1. Marriage--Religious aspects--Orthodox Eastern Church–Congresses. 2. Family--Religious life--Congresses. 3. Medicine--Religious aspects--Orthodox Eastern Church--Congresses. 4. Psychology and religion –Congresses. 5. Christianity--Psychology--Congresses. 6. Orthodox Eastern Church--Doctrines--Congresses. 7. Greek Orthodox Archdiocese of North and South America–Doctrines--Congresses. I. Chirban, John T. II. Symposium on Medicine, psychology, religion. 1983. IV. Series. [DNLM: 1. Marriage--Congresses. 2. Family--Congresses. HQ 728 M359]
BX378.M2M37 1983 261.8'358 83-22526
ISBN 0-916586-63-4

Marriage and the Family

Medicine, Psychology and Religion:

New Directions, New Integrations

CONTENTS

INTRODUCTION

The series on Medicine, Psychology and Religion is an outgrowth of the annual symposium on Medicine, Psychology and Religion. This colloquium was inaugurated to provide a forum for Greek and Orthodox professionals to share with one another their approaches in human service.

The purpose for the annual programs is to establish a gathering between medicine, psychology and religion. Although we are hoping to learn about the content of one and another's discipline, the accent of this venture is to appreciate how we may work together to help the people that we serve.

This interdisciplinary dialogue works to offer insight into the contemporary concerns of Greek people and Orthodox Christians. The primary objective of these meetings is to unite and to share interests among friends in the human services. Therefore, the symposia are not specifically intended to be scholarly exchanges.

The Symposium on "Marriage and the Family" had two purposes: First, to explore the relationship and compatability of the fields of psychology and religion, which will be of ongoing concern for the symposia; and, second, to present psychological and theological perspectives on the particular topic of this day, "Marriage and the Family."

The Symposium on "Medicine, Psychology and Religion: New Directions and New Integrations" provided an opportunity for a physician, theologian and pastoral psychologist to discuss the interdependency of these disciplines from three perspectives.

INTRODUCTION

This publication represents the substance of the formal presentations of the day. It serves as a ledger of the annual meetings. Through the continued interest of the Greek Orthodox Archdiocese, Hellenic College and the Hellenic Counseling Association these dialogues and this publication will continue.

The joint Symposia Committee of the sponsoring organizations included Reverend Alkiviades C. Calivas, Dr. John T. Chirban, Reverend George Economou, Dr. Arthur Pappas, Ms. Carol Senopoulos, Ms. Elaine Seteropoulos and Ms. Eve Welts.

I wish to express sincere appreciation to Dr. Thomas C. Lelon, president of Hellenic College and Holy Cross School of Theology, for his strong, personal encouragement of the Symposium and to express appreciation for the support of Hellenic College, which hosted the annual meetings. I also wish to cite the careful and patient assistance of Marcia Hetman who typed the manuscripts of this publication and to acknowledge the Reverend Dr. Nomikos Vaporis for guiding the printing of this publication.

The Editor

I. MARRIAGE AND THE FAMILY

THE DIALOGUE OF PSYCHOLOGY AND THEOLOGY

by John T. Chirban

Mental health workers and the clergy have long been grouped together as "helping professionals." But does much of a relationship exist between them? Are their services similar? Should one go to a psychiatrist or to a priest in the turmoil of marital or family problems? Would the advice of these different professionals lead to diametrically opposed conclusions? Or would the differences be insignificant?

My task today is to speak about the interaction of psychology and theology. I will address the questions: What are the basic similarities and differences between psychology and theology? Can there really be a dialogue between these disciplines? And, if so, how can a dialogue occur?

The apprehension and enmity between these fields is common knowledge. Actually psychology and religion have rarely shared peace. An article in last month's **Boston Globe** reflects the tension. There, "the fact" was stated that psychiatrists experience the subject of religion as "taboo in therapy" since "people perceive psychiatrists . . . in competition with the clergy."

Dr. John T. Chirban is Chairman of the Department of Human Development and Director of the Office of Counseling and Guidance at Hellenic College and Holy Cross School of Theology. He is an Associate in Human Development at Harvard University and maintains a private practice in psychotherapy in Cambridge, Massachusetts.

Well are they? To be honest, I feel much trepidation as I stand before you, an audience with mixed and possibly competitive backgrounds: students and teachers; laymen and clergy; patients and doctors; theologians and psychologists/psychiatrists; churched and unchurched.

Can such diversified groups really hear one another? Before addressing this question, let's examine how mental health and religious professionals have met and understood one another. To do this, I will provide a brief summary of what has been said about psychology and religion.

I. WHAT HAS BEEN SAID ABOUT PSYCHOLOGY AND RELIGION:

As I have examined the literature concerning the dialogue between psychology and religion, the **single** fact that impressed me was that while many things have been said, these discussions have often seemed fragmented, partial or diffuse. For example, there is a considerable amount of writing about the "differences of psychology and religion."

A. THE DIFFERENCES OF PSYCHOLOGY AND RELIGION

It is not uncommon to read about the general similarities of and differences between psychology and religion. Drawing upon many of the studies, one might deduce the following matrix:

	PSYCHOLOGY	**RELIGION**
FOUNDATION	Scientific	Theological
PHILOSOPHY	Anthropocentric	Theocentric
SPIRIT	Secular	Sacred
APPROACH	Self-Correcting	Dogmatic
ATTITUDE	Dispassionate	Committed

Although there are kernels of truth to these characterizations, in addition to polarizing the fields and churning emotional and often defensive reactions, such generalizations do not seem helpful after serious examination. In fact, there are significant problems with these claims. For example:

1. **Regarding the claim that Psychology and Religion have, respectively, Scientific or Theological Foundations:**

To state that it is solely psychology which uses the scientific method blurs our awareness of the fact that there are implicit "theologies" or assumptions about the nature of the person behind all personality theories. Certainly "objective" science itself professes an inherent philosophy. Also, to characterize religion as having only theological foundations is to forget that religion is shaped by methods of human beings, on the one hand, including the strengths of the scientific method, and, on the other hand, the interpretations of the individual "theologian."

2. **Regarding the claim that Psychology and Religion have, respectively, Anthropocentric or Theocentric Perspectives:**

To generalize about anthropocentric and theocentric qualities of psychology and religion is to suggest psychology and religion present two distinct perspectives rather than to acknowledge the fact that psychology and religion are, independently, very broad fields with at least as many opposing as complementary positions within each area. Further, within each discipline one may identify approaches that are more or less anthropocentric or theocentric.

3. **Regarding the claim that Psychology and Religion are, respectively, Secular or Sacred:**

To polarize psychology and religion as secular versus sacred is to obscure the reality that both fields reflect human and divine experiences and interventions. And although psychology may be presented as overtly **descriptive** and theology as clearly **prescriptive,** a closer examination of the fields evidences at minimum the inherent prescriptions in **psychology** and implicit descriptions of **theology.**

4. **Regarding the claim that Psychology and Religion are, respectively, Self-Correcting or Dogmatic:**

To perceive psychology as self-correcting and religion as dogmatic reflects a loss of historical perspective. In the case of religion, the history of the church demonstrates accommodation and changes in the presentation of the Message of the times. And, in the case of psychology, to perceive the field as basically self-correcting ignores the reality that numerous stubborn, dogmatic positions determine, in fact, what the schools of psychology are all about.

5. **Regarding the claim that Psychology and Religion are, respectively, Dispassionate or Committed:**

It has been common to stereotype that psychologists emphasize a distant, clinical approach to life and that theologians express a personal, caring approach in their work. Although these characterizations may, in part, be accurate, when they are predominate styles they skew the power of these disciplines. In fact, when psychology and theology balance both a committed and dispassionate approach they are most effective.

In the final analysis, such generalizations have resulted in creating significant gaps, but have not offered any clarification pertaining to the similarities and differences or to the constructive understanding concerning the relationship between psychology and religion. What of the dialogue then? Are we to be left with an ill-defined subject? Can we not offer any more clarity to this discussion? Let us consider what clinical and mental health professionals themselves say:

B. SURVEY OF MENTAL HEALTH AND RELIGIOUS PROFESSIONALS

A recent article in a Boston newspaper reported the results of an informal survey of area psychologists, psychiatrists and clergy about the interfacing roles of clergy and mental health professionals. The findings revealed these diverse impressions:

1. From the Psychological Perspective:

It was stated that many pastors were thought as ill-prepared to deal with anything more than "a nagging spiritual crisis." One psychologist said, " . . . clergy do not distinguish someone who is suffering from a psychotic depression over and against a simple disappointment."

Certainly the range of views differed. Psychotherapists evaluated the skills of clergy from: "It's sort of like people who talk to their hairdresser" to " . . . it is nothing less than the clergy's sworn duty to tinker with its parishioners' emotional ailments." One psychologist humbly stated, "There's a tendency among psychiatrists and psychologists to exaggerate in an extreme way the amount of skills they have. They often overrate their effectiveness and underrate the effectiveness and intelligence of other professionals."

2. From the Religious Perspective:

A clergywoman stated that the nonclinical relationship between minister and parishioner **is** compatible with the counseling process and precludes the "I'm nuts" stigma often identified with therapy. She said, "I can help a lot of people who feel talking to me is not threatening, but the idea of a shrink is devastating."

One clergyman, however, pointed out the need for religious counselors to be clearly differentiated from therapists as "complications arise because of the conflicting roles."

From this summary, we see that a dialogue between psychology and religion does not occur between two distinct positions. In fact, the interface between psychology and religion seems to have unclear boundaries being ill-defined and emotionally charged - - involving issues of territoriality, biases and multiple ways of thinking about the disciplines. So, is there a way to order the situation? Can there really be a dialogue?

II. MODELS FOR A DIALOGUE

As I sorted through the literature, I thought that the most heuristic approach to trying to understand the relationship between the disciplines of psychology and religion is to examine how people **think** about them. Since we are concerned with bridging communications between psychology and religion, I thought it would be helpful to try to identify ways in which we think about these fields - - that is, how we conceptualize the discussion - - to clarify the structure of our thought. So, I will describe stages here, not as in a formal theory of structural developmental thought, but as in approaches that I have witnessed and experienced in my study of this field.[1]

In accordance with our time limitations, I will briefly introduce the stages of these models, and I will provide examples of psychologists and theologians who reflect the characterizations of the models. This presentation does not intend to identify all the possible models, but seeks to make the point that there are different ways that people **think** about psychology and religion. Communication between the disciplines will be facilitated as people become clear about their own thinking and as they engage in the dialogue as well as become open to the approaches of others.

Although psychology and religion are represented in the following discussions as units, I want to acknowledge, again, that both fields separately include a variety of perspectives, often conflicting with

---

[1] I have built on the work of my mentor, Dr. William R. Rogers, in considering models for a dialogue (See William R. Rogers, "The Dynamics of Psychology and Religion: Teaching in a Dialogical Field," Society for the Scientific Study of Religion, Annual Meeting, Chicago, October, 1977.)

one another. In the diagrams of stages the solid circle represents the issue or phenomenon under discussion; e.g., a person with anxiety. The vertical line is the direction of analysis; the "Ψ" (ψυχολογία) indicates a psychological evaluation; the "Θ" (θεολογία) indicates a religious evaluation; the "A" (ἀλήθεια) represents Truth.

TERMS

In this discussion, psychology (ψηχολογία) is defined as the modern scientific study of behavior. Religion refers to the system of faith of the individual. Religion (θρησκεία) rather than "theology" (θεολογία) is translated here from the Greek. I reserve the term theology as "the expeience of God," and, in so doing, understand that it may occur even outside of religion. "Theology" is discussed in the last model. Note, however, that the terms theological and religion are used interchangeably in the discussion of models. Truth (᾿Αλήθεια) here refers to the Ultimate Truth.

As we review the following eight models of dialogue, ask yourself which paradigm best characterizes your approach to the interdisciplinary discussion. Also, consider whether or not you have observed the other perspectives. Most important, ask yourself if the style which characterizes your approach to this dialogue is truest to your interest and ask how well it serves your intents.

As we review these models, I will reflect on how I have witnessed these approaches in my life, and I will provide examples of theorists whose works demonstrate the basic thrusts of these perspectives.

1. **Monolithic Model**

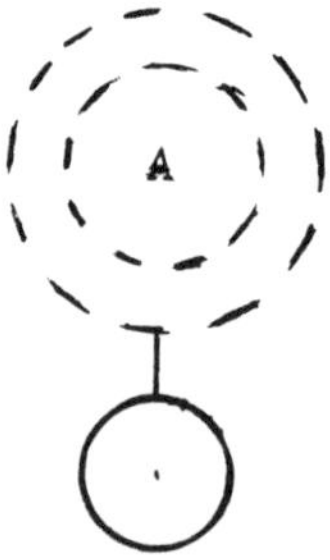

The monolithic model may reflect either a psychological or a theological understanding. One of the distinctive features of this perspective is that it is basically egocentric. The egocentricity is experienced by how one is either uninformed or totally indifferent to views other than his own. From this model, all of life can be interpreted according to either a psychological or theological vision. Material not made immediately clear through the particular approach is left unattended. This view is like that of a young child who sees only through his own eyes.

This perspective, however, may be represented by psychologists or theologians who fail to take seriously the role of the "other" discipline in life. Such individuals fail to acknowledge the existence of other perspectives and seem to need to explain all of life from their own vantage points. This results in a myopic and imperialistic vision.

2. **Beclouded Model**

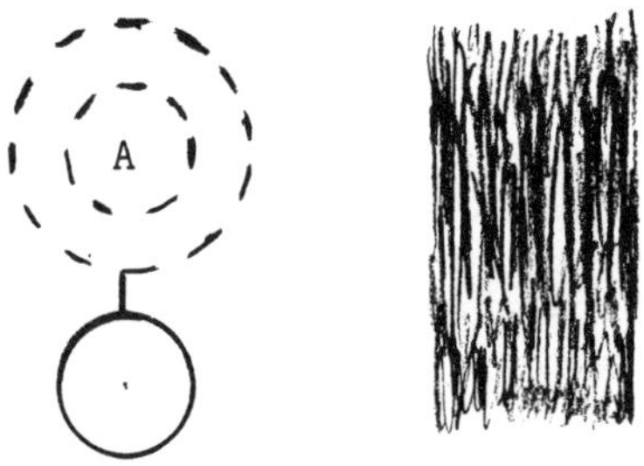

This model differs from the earlier conceptual framework in that it knows that there are other perspectives. The individual in this case, however, does not clearly understand what is out there. This approach is shared by those who know that there are perspectives about life different than their own but who are not clear about the specific details of the differences - - neither what they are nor what they say - - much less the way in which the "other" perspective interacts with the particular individual's perception of a phenomenon.

I can recall thinking in this way during my high school years, before my senior course in psychology. At the time, I understood all things only according to my commitments to the Orthodox Christian faith. I had simply heard of this "psychology" - - which heretofore I did not understand. For me the area held credibility only because an academic course was designed for its study. What it had to say and how it affected me was this "clouded mystery." For all practical purposes, it was undifferentiated and outside of my immediate environment and needs.

3. **Polarized Model**

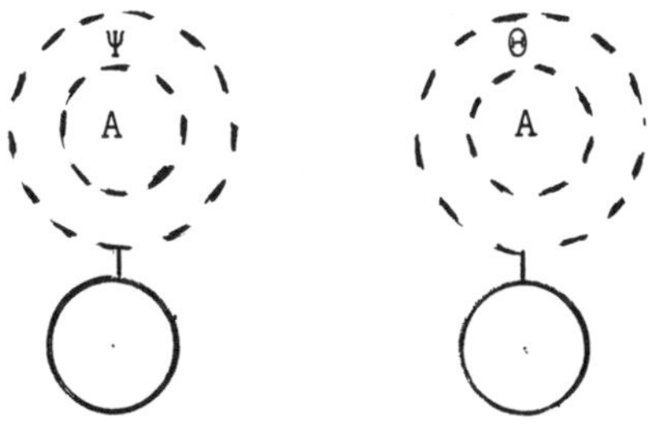

The polarized model clearly acknowledges and presents psychology and religion as being concerned with two opposing ranges of phenomena. The polarization is between their approaches - - much like the distinctions that I identified in the earlier discussion of similarities and differences: Scientific vs. Theological; Anthropocentric vs. Theocentric; Secular vs. Sacred, etc. Here, psychology, for example, may understand religion as a reality but may treat it as a learned set of behavior; and religion may understand psychology as a useful discipline but may relegate its role to treating the "fallen nature of humanity."

After my first course in psychology, the polarization model seemed to provide me with a helpful way of managing what seemed to be two different approaches to human beings. This way of thinking provided me with a way to categorize and even to stereotype the functions of the disciplines. It enabled me to acknowledge conveniently the importance of psychology and religion as well as providing a method of avoiding the more complex aspects of life which were "grey" by placing them in this "either/or" matrix.

It was here, at Hellenic College, that the polarization model did not seem adequate to accomodate my new concerns. At that time I was introduced to behaviorism in a course of college psychology. I found that the position of B. F. Skinner, with his presupposition of determinism, could not be rectified honestly by my polarization model. More specifically, the philosophical issues that Skinner raised did not fit into the psychological part of this model. This created much tension and unrest within me. What to do with the dissonance? Well, I approached my spiritual father for help. After much discussion, he suggested that I read Skinner's work directly and that we should talk further. He wisely perceived that this was a growing edge for me. That summer, I worked in the morning as a security guard in Chicago. And with a gun that I really did not know how to shoot, in one hand, and with one of Skinner's books in the other hand, I intensely read through the pages yearning to rectify my confusion. I scrupulously prepared notes from my readings and worked through the issues with my spiritual father over the phone in conversations to Boston which would take place during the night.

After many conversations with my spiritual father, I finally mustered the nerve to pose my burning, bottom-line question. "So," I asked, "what if Skinner is right? What if determinism is "the truth" and there is "no choice?" To this he calmly answered, "If Skinner is right then religion is poetry. But," he added, "the issue remains whether or not he is correct. This is something that you will have to decide for yourself." And so we move to the next model.

4. **Reductionistic Model**

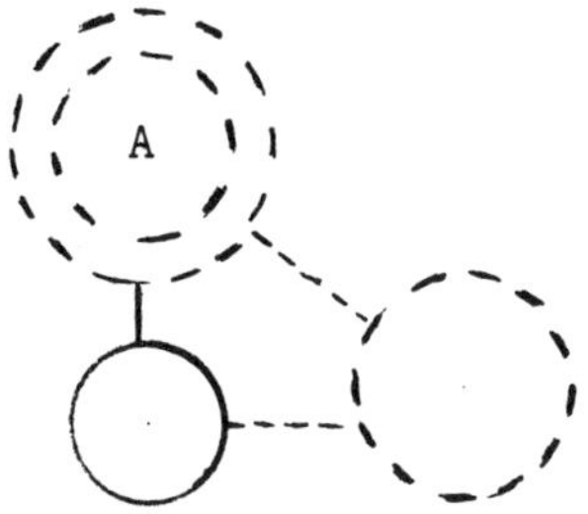

The reductionistic model dilutes the "other" position through prejudicial evaluations and lack of serious attentiveness to the other's perspective. Functionally, this position maintains that the Truth is available only to its own constituency. Both psychology and religion have been guilty of this approach - - which is, in large measure, the reason for the tension that exists between them. Two cases in point:

Although it would not be accurate to characterize Sigmund Freud and B. F. Skinner in this way, in every detail, nevertheless, they have done the most to fuel the psychological reductionistic perspective.

For Freud, religious practice and belief is prompted essentially by neurotic and psychotic motivation. He speaks specifically of religion in terms of obsessive and compulsive traits, illusion and delusion; wish fulfillment and unresolved Oedipal striving; the return of repressed guilt and "infantile patterns of helplessness" - - in addition to projection and displacement.

And for Skinner, religion is discussed and understood basically as a "mode of control." For him, the teachings about heaven and hell epitomize the use of positive and negative reinforcement. Heaven and hell, he states, provide the foundation of religious power.

Most of us would agree that "religious activity," in particular instances, may exhibit traits of these analyses, but we would not present these perspectives exclusively as representing the motives or functions of religion. In both instances, here, the psychoanalytic and behavioristic perspectives clearly reduce the intrinsic value of religion.

During my graduate work, I had the opportunity to discuss these concerns with B. F. Skinner, in terms of what I call here the "psychological reductionistic approach" between psychology and religion.[2]

In that discussion, Skinner explained the purpose of religion as he saw it:

> I would like to see religion permit one to examine the world, study it scientifically, without any threat that one is going to counter to reveal truth. My own belief about God is that we are on a very small planet around a mediocre sun, which is one of billions of suns in our own galaxy and there are billions of galaxies. Now if God created all of that, who the devil are we to know anything about Him? I think it's ridiculous to suppose we can know God, and I don't see why God should reveal anything to us.

From this statement, it was evident to me that Skinner maintains an epistemology which precludes the experience of God. So I asked him, "Can there be other ways of being religious and experiencing God that are not explained through power and control - - but through prayer?"[3] To this he responded, "Well, if God revealed Himself to us in the many different ways reported by different religions, and if I choose one, I would obviously choose one because of my culture, my own history." In saying this, the limits of Skinner's approach to the dialogue of psychology and religion are clearly drawn.

It should be noted that this same model may be witnessed inversely by the religious reductionistic perspective. Theologians who represent this approach may express defensive, sweeping generalities about psychiatry and psychology. They envision the Truth as accessible to religion alone and relegate the psychological disciplines to being faithless, secular and unnecessary. In addition to ignoring the fact that inspired, positive roles of religion have been affirmed by psychologists such as Jung, James and Allport, the individuals

---

[2]I conducted a number of interviews with B. F. Skinner which addressed topics of motivation, philosophy and religion in terms of behaviorism. Currently, I am completing a book in collaboration with Dr. Skinner about behaviorism and religion.

[3]This question emerges from Kant, who states that it is impossible for the natural (man) to know the supernatural (God) except by supernatural means. Kant suggests that God provides the supernatural medium through prayer thereby linking man and God.

represented in this model express a narrow, possessive attitude which suggests that they have the final hold on the Truth. They see little importance in work outside of their own sphere and they are closed to the truth that is available to other perspectives.

Whether the reductionistic model is maintained by psychology or religion, this approach purports to be all-pervasive and comprehensive. Needless to say, it precludes an interactive, investigative or collegial approach.

5. **Corrective Model**

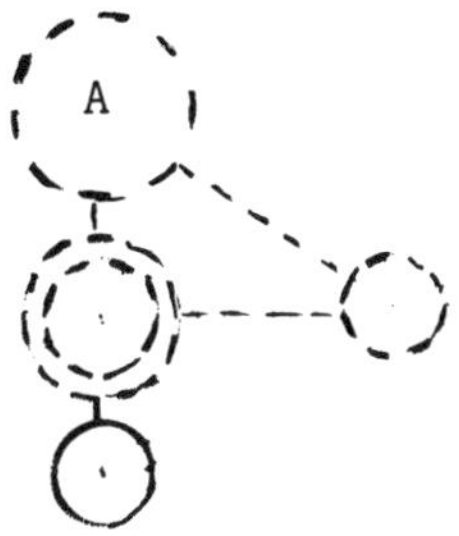

The corrective model attends to the value of the "other" perspective but has primary commitment to its own purposes. From the diagram, we may describe the discipline that is in line vertically (with a double dotted circle) as the **primary** discipline (either psychology or theology) and the dotted circle to the right as the secondary discipline.

When religion is in the vertical position, the primary analysis is theological. Additional insights from the psychological side are heard - - but, finally, a religious evaluation is offered. In this case, the bias is that religion provides the more penetrating analysis of the two. One witnesses this model frequently in pastoral psychological literature.

This does not have to be the case, but writers in pastoral psychology who work in this way do not often describe their purposes which, in the final analysis, bring the religious perspective in the limelight. This approach is also experienced by mental health professionals who do not understand religion. Although they discuss faith, their primary allegiance is to a psychological evaluation.

One observes that in this model the particular **discipline** - - not the dialogue - - is primary. Usually, the secondary discipline is analyzed in the interest of the primary discipline. In doing this, obviously the secondary discipline is presented as having less importance.

Although somewhat dialogical, the model clearly reflects a one-upmanship: there appears to be an investment by "promoters" of this model and a need for the "primary discipline" to reign.

6. **Dialogical Model**

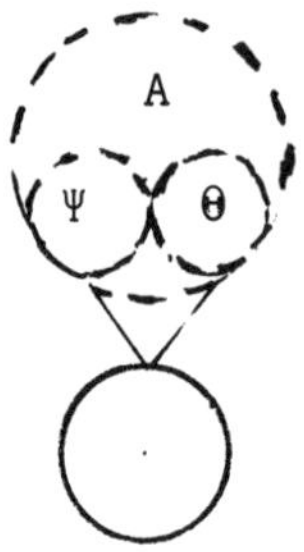

The dialogical model attempts to open a fair communication between psychology and religion. It affirms the inherent value in both psychology and religion and seeks to facilitate communication between these perspectives as they attend to human situations.

Like the polarized model, however, there often remains the perception that psychology attends to pathology and religion to moral health. However, another, more critical problem is that this model, as presented by psychologists or theologians, tends to overlook or to neglect the particular implicit methodological problems or unique contributions offered by psychology and by religion. In the effort to encourage the dialogue, therefore, important discriminations are not made. The boundaries of the disciplines are taken lightly or are not discussed.

Efforts like those of Ernest Becker, on Denial and Finitude, or John Kornarakes, on the Orthodox Tradition and Modern Psychology, are cases in point. Although enlightening, these works do not give adequate attention to the methodology and commitments of the issues which they address.

7. **Theoretical Model**

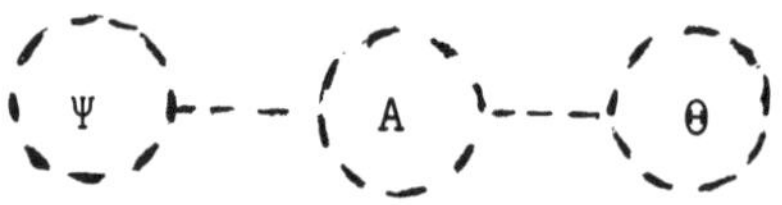

[5]See Peter Homans, The Dialogue Between Psychology and Religion (Chicago: University of Chicago Press, 1968), which presents numerous essays reflecting this model.

The theoretical model is offered as "a goal" by people who speak about the values for interdisciplinary work between psychology and religion. This model is less than an approach to the dialogue as it tends to lack discussions of concrete phenomena. It is theoretical, but not empirical. It represents more an **abstract** enterprise than a substantive dialogue through affirming the **principles** of a genuine dialogue between psychology and religion.

Elhard's work is demonstrative of this approach, where features of what he calls "pervasiveness, relationship, tension, charge, identification and diffusion" are presented as common structures in psychology and religion. Heavy theoretical language is present with little or no empirical or practicable discussion.

The theoretical model works to consider seriously the aspects of a dialogue for psychology and religion. It is concerned with the methodological details and specific problems of each discipline. The discussion, however, is by theoretical abstraction and obviates the needs to consider both real situations and meaningful dialogues.

8. **Dynamic Model**

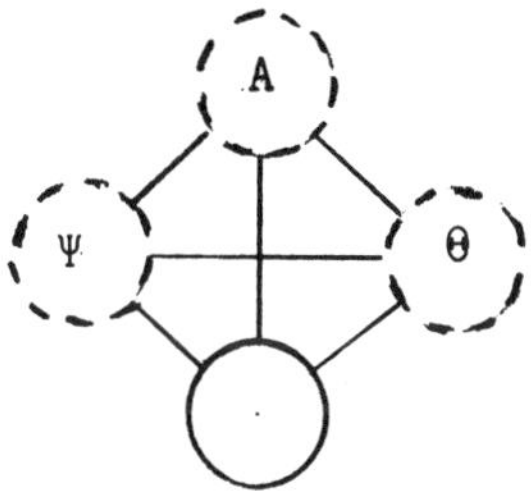

The dynamic model is concerned with the boundaries, methods and tasks of both psychology and religion and attends to their content and implications as they relate to one's life experience.

This model identifies the Truth as accessible to both disciplines as well as to the individual. Certainly, no corner on Truth is suggested by this perspective. The approach maintains the strengths of the disciplines and engages one in a genuine dialogue. Differences are noted, not hidden. The resonant qualities of the disciplines are presented and affirmed. The dynamic model encourages a critical, serious relationship between psychology and religion.

The dynamic model shows that the solutions to problems need not be understood from one or the other approaches, psychology or religion alone but, ideally, may draw upon the resources of both disciplines. It is the most balanced and objective approach to the dialogue that I will describe.

ORTHODOX CHRISTIAN APPROACH

In the time remaining, I wish to say a few words concerning the dialogue of psychology and religion for Orthodox Christian faith vis a vis the models that I have presented. I suggest that the Orthodox Christian approach to the dialogue should be an attempt to relate the interests of modern psychology and theology in the spirit of the Doctors of the Orthodox Christian faith. This, I believe, may be accomplished through the dynamic model.

Up until this time I have not clarified my usage of the terms "religion" and "theology." We know that Orthodox **theology** is defined as the **experience** of God, as differentiated from theological **discussion** or abstractions. At the same time, it is recognized that Orthodox Christianity is also experienced as a **religion**, with an accent on the **institutional activity** that may not be part of "the experiencing of God." Thc challenge of our particular tradition is to reflect the Truth of God through experiencing Him to the greatest degree possible. The purpose of this distinction, here, is to emphasize that Orthodox Christianity is truth according to the degree to which it reflects the experience of God. Orthodoxy cannot be threatened by a dynamic dialogue with psychology because, by definition, Orthodoxy is the True Teaching. Clearly that Teaching is not limited to one discipline. The dynamic model is valuable in that it clarifies the fact that there are not only different kinds of knowing - - e.g., physiological, psychological or theological - - but, finally, that there is one Truth. The dynamic model frees us from the temptation to think that we can control the Truth.

In summary, this presentation has focused upon how people think in the dialogue of psychology and religion. Other perspectives also may be offered. One notes, in the models which have been discussed, that there is a progression towards bridging the gap between the analyst's couch and the church's pew. As we progress from the monolithic model to the dynamic model, suspicion and hostility are replaced by communication, affirmation and mutual support - - reflective of the ultimate value of love and the reality that the human being is fullest as a psycho-somatic unity. In this way, the dynamic model nurtures good health of mind and soul.

The disciplines of psychology and religion offer much to modern times through their particular insights and perspectives. By drawing nearer to one another it is emphasized that their power is magnified. Both mental health professionals and religious leaders have observed what our "divided selves" have yielded, what one priest calls "the fears of nothingness, the horror of emptiness" - - or lack of faith - - and what a motivational psychologist refers to as "existential sickness"- -or having no meaning. In the final analysis, the advances of our times are leading helping professionals to work together towards assisting humankind to be not fragmented but whole.

MAINTAINING GREEK AND ORTHODOX IDENTITY IN AMERICA

THEOLOGICAL PERSPECTIVE

by James C. Christon

The concept of "maintaining" an identity is a complex one; it suggests that what already exists should be retained without further consideration. I'm not at all sure this idea is valid for our times. In fact, I strongly suspect that it is not. Moreover, the concept doesn't answer the question: "If an identity ought to me maintained, **which** identity should that be?"

Everyone, I presume, is aware of the need for identity from a sociological as well as a psychological point of view. As an individual's self-awareness emerges, the need to develop a clear sense of identity correlates with the developing self. In fact, for Erik Erikson, identity is a central developmental task. To have a clearly defined sense of self is supreme. He states:

> The identity of the adolescent seeks to clarify who he is, what his role is in society, and what the role is to be. Is he a child or is he an adult? Does he have it in him

---

Reverend James C. Christon is Pastor of "The Assumption" Greek Orthodox Church in Manchester, New Hampshire. He is Instructor of Social Sciences and Psychology at River College and Hesser College. He is also a Visiting Lecturer at Notre Dame College.

> someday to be a husband and father? What is he to be as a worker or an earner of money? Can he feel confident in spite of the fact that his race or religion or national background make him a person some people look down upon? Overall, will he be a success or a failure?

While the foregoing refers to an individual and an adolescent in search of the self, notwithstanding, this is also true of an organization such as a Church. The same pressing need arises - - the need to identify properly itself to itself and to others. This will be paramount to its acceptance in society.

The formation of a stable sense of identity is not an easy task for any entity - - individual or organizational. Rapid physical and social changes that confuse the continuity between the past and the present only make the task more difficult. Like most people who suffer from role confusion and fail to establish a clear identity, social and political organizations such as the Church, which exist to support the formulation of such an identity, also suffer in the quest to define themselves and their purpose.

The family, which has long been an important part of the Church's social identity, is presently in crisis. Values long associated with family life - - permanent union, kinship, loyalty, motherhood - - to name just a few - - are losing their previously unquestioned and absolute character. The role of the extended family has been undermined by excessive emphasis on the nuclear family unit. The authority of the parent has eroded, even though this originally aided the child to identify with the family unit. A sense of family identity in the broad sense has dissipated, and the very necessity for family organization is being seriously challenged.

This identity crisis of the family has in turn affected the Church's identity. For the Church is nothing more than the continuance of the family concept in the sense that it is a family under the fatherhood of God. Perhaps the most important question psychology deals with - - the question of identity, of "who am I?" - - is also the most important question facing the Church today.

Seventy-five years or more have passed since Orthodoxy first appeared on the American scene. During that time, we, as an ecclesiastical entity, have struggled to define and present a meaningful ecclesiastical image - - an image that can be universally understood and accepted.

As I stressed before, each of us as people needs to establish our own separate identities: each individual needs that special element that accents his or her uniqueness. Our own personal names set us apart - - one from another. In the same way we are set apart as Christians. In St. Paul's words, "Ye are peculiar," we recognize a reference to the uniqueness that is ours. The Book of Acts refers to those who chose Christianity as "Followers of the Way." Every reference places a special uniqueness on us. As Greek Orthodox we add yet another term that speaks to a special identity - - the word, "Greek."

For all too long we have accepted the myth of the "melting pot" of America. This was the theory, as you know, that supposedly referred to the eventual complete assimilation of ethnic groups into the mainstream of American society. Our forefathers, in their efforts to assimilate tried desperately to dilute their true identity in order to conform to the social demands of the dominant group. They shortened or anglicized their names. They strove to learn the language and integrate the culture of America into their lives. They endeavored to join through whatever means the mainstream of society. They joined organizations, associations, clubs and de-emphasized their religious and ethnic differences. At first the identity crisis tended to be overwhelming; concessions were made at the greater expense of the self. What they eventually learned from all their efforts was the futility of them. To give up an identity leaves a person in a psychological social vacuum. The individual is left without a clear-cut definition of who he or she is.

Ecclesiastically, we also tried - - at great length I might add - -to provide some semblance to other Churches, in an attempt to de-emphasize our own uniqueness. Our theology adopted terms, nomenclature, if you will, and concepts entirely foreign to our dogmatic and theological positions. Remnants of this attempt are still with us.

But apparently the real image, the true identity of the Orthodox Church in the Americas continues to elude us. Who indeed are we? What is Orthodoxy? Even among Orthodox groups we see "57 varieties" - - tendencies to accent positions, names contradictory to the real pursuit of the Faith we espouse. Moreover, confusion reigns supreme in the attempt to fuse our ethnic identities with the unadulterated concept of the Church - - suggesting to the innocent bystander that membership in Greek Orthodoxy apparently demands a Greek ethnic heritage. We baptize converts and hear our people refer to "making a Greek out of them" - - or "they were married in a Greek Church," whatever that is supposed to mean. We even have backlash, within the Church from those who speak of a purely "American Orthodox Church." This causes a rent in relations between those who under God should be closest.

If identity is so important - - and we can agree it is - - then our strongest desire should be to identify and be identified properly. Are we Greek? or Greek Orthodox? Are we Russian or Russian Orthodox? Such distinctions may be questioned ad infinitum as we consider the varied ethnic groups that constitute world Orthodoxy. Or should our main pursuit be to establish a single religious identity more encompassing than an ethnic appellation might suggest?

History shows that historians and theologians alike rarely make ethnic distinctions in referring to Orthodoxy, but rather, relate to the oneness of Faith either by speaking of Orthodoxy or the Eastern Church (as distinct from the Roman Catholic or Western Church). Would this be more preferable? Or would those who want ethnic emphasis feel excluded?

In my opinion, this issue will continue to plague the Church as a divisive issue that hinders the establishment of a true identity of Orthodoxy. Furthermore, it confuses our people. Stability of the personality is impossible unless an answer to the serious question posed at the beginning of this presentation is forthcoming.

Identity we need. But it must be well thought out. We must find that identity to which each of us singularly and as a group can properly relate. We must tenaciously avoid superficialities that more than not undermine the very intent and meaningfulness of identity itself.

I once again return to the initial question - - what is it we wish to maintain? Prior to any consideration of this point, it is essential that we must first **define the identity** that is Orthodoxy.

MAINTAINING GREEK AND ORTHODOX IDENTITY IN AMERICA

PSYCHOLOGICAL PERSPECTIVE

by John C. Papajohn

This past Easter Day I talked to an old man. He was, in spite of his years, physically strong, with a robust frame and clear blue eyes that sparkled as he talked. The sparkle reinforced the general enthusiasm he manifested in our conversation about his immigration to the United States from Greece more than sixty years ago. He was fourteen years old when he had come alone from his village near Sparta, Greece. He had wanted to come for a long time and finally prevailed over the protestations of his father and mother who were afraid that they would never see him again. He came, buoyed by the adventure of it all, and joined a cousin in a midwestern state. There he began his career as a shoe-shine boy. He worked hard, learned his trade well and soon opened his own shoe-shine shop and expanded the services he offered his customers to include, among other things, the block pressing of their hats.

Now sixty years later, we stood in the living room of his daughter's home. It was a large and luxuriously furnished home. My friend

---

Dr. John Papajohn maintains a private practice in psychotherapy in Brookline, Massachusetts. He consults at Cambridge City Hospital, Boston's Veterans' Administration Hospital and Hellenic College. He is the author of Transactions in Families with John Spiegel, published by Jossey-Bass, and another book about behavior therapy which is soon to be published by Pergamon Press.

was manifestly proud of the achievements of his son-in-law who was a prominent businessman in the community in which they lived. He was also proud of his grandchildren and their children who circulated through the house as is typical in Greek homes where the Resurrection is feted with much joy on Easter Day. And when I asked my friend to tell me about those original Greeks who had come to the United States, wondering aloud about their determination to succeed in the New World, he responded with two phrases that shall always remain with me. We had **potho** he said and "we cared about each other." Now **potho** has a two fold meaning: it means "desire" but it also means "hope." I want to share with you some thoughts about this **potho** of our fathers and I also want to talk to you about the other characteristic of theirs - - their ability to care for one another. These, I feel, are the two most important gifts they have given and I often grieve when I feel we may be losing them.

It was the "desire" and "hope" for a better life that motivated our fathers to leave their villages, their farms, their flocks and their families to come to the New World. In this regard they did not differ from those who had come before them in waves of immigration that reached back to the original pilgrims themselves. Our fathers, however, in contrast to the original American settlers, did not leave their country to find freedom from religious and political persecution. They came, instead, because America offered the promise of providing the resources to create a better life for themselves and their families. America provided the opportunity but it was in their native Greece that their individual aspirations and dreams were born and nurtured. The essence of this "desire" and this "hope" emanated from the strong pervasive sense of national consciousness that has always been a central feature of Greek culture. Greeks have always loved their country. This love, which has been expressed through fierce loyalty and through the sacrifice of much blood over the ages is the foundation on which their individual pride, their sense of personal dignity - - indeed, the meaning of being itself - - is based. It is the source that nourishes their "desire" and "hope" for the attainment of individual excellence and individual achievement. This has always been the "Greek way." The achievements of their ancestors from the fifth century B.C. and before, to the present are for them a continuing wellspring of "desire" and "hope." A Greek identifies himself first in terms of his country. He is bound to his countrymen by the strong ties of a shared heritage that has a real and immediate presence for him regardless of where in the world he may find himself. Greeks "care for one another." It is in this caring that their existence finds meaning.

And so when my old friend and his friends came to this country, it was not to escape the subjugation and injustices of the old country, as was the case with the original immigrants and many who came later. They did not come to find freedom from the values and ways of the "old country." They came instead to realize themselves through the expression of the same values in the form of a strong determination to excell and to succeed through the expression of their individualism in a new country that promised to provide them with the resources to do so.

But when our fathers arrived on these shores, the "native" Americans who were their hosts did not at first discern these values and these aspirations of the new immigrants from the values and aspirations of immigrants from southern Europe. They saw dark and swarthy men and women who spoke another one of those "peasant languages," who clustered together in the poorer sections of the cities and who were willing to fill the ranks of the laborers who were sorely needed to work in the factories and on the railroads in a period of great economic growth. They also worked as shoe-shine boys, like my friend, and dishwashers and waiters in the restaurants of those "host" Americans who had arrived in this country before them. They worked hard in these menial occupations and were grateful for the opportunity. Greeks, however, cannot be content for long to work for others. In the villages from which they had come they owned their own plot of land, they were their own bosses; they could not find it easy to subject themselves to anyone. And so in this country they soon owned their own hot-dog carts, and popcorn stands and then their own restaurants. They saved their money and bought their own shoe-shine shops like my old friend did in his youth; they bought florist shops and other small businesses and entered gradually into the mainstream of American entrepreneurship.

Their "host" American friends looked favorably on this activity of these new immigrants. They were good family people and good citizens. They were adjusting to the American way of life; they were becoming "good Americans." The "host" Americans did not know that, in fact, these new immigrants were expressing what was for them the "Greek way of life." They were not adapting to new cultural forms in this new land; they were not changing their way of life to conform to the expectations of their American hosts. They were being Greeks as Greeks have always been in different parts of the world and in all times. They were realizing their individual aspirations to excel and to achieve the most that they could for themselves and for their children. They were expressing their **potho** for a better life and they were doing it in American terms. There was no other way.

But there was another aspect of the Greek way of life in the United States that was not understood as well as their economic activity was: this was the habit that Greeks had of sticking together and limiting their social contacts to other Greeks. They quickly established their churches wherever they went and these became the centers of their communities. On Sundays, they gathered together to celebrate the Liturgy and also to celebrate Greek Independence Day and other special days that marked important events in the country they had come from. All of this did not seem very American at all.

What the "host" Americans did not know, however, was that the Greek community provided the social form through which these new immigrants renewed themselves by the continued maintenance of their sense of ethnic consciousness. They reaffirmed each Sunday "who" they were. They reaffirmed their common Hellenism which strengthened them individually and kept alive their desire and their hope for a better tomorrow in the new world to which they had come. They also renewed in their coming together the caring that they felt for one another. During the week they worked hard at their jobs or in their businesses for long hours. On Sundays they were reunited with great joy. It was here in the Greek community that they could really be themselves; relax, talk about the old country and about friends and relatives in other parts of America. It was the spontaneity of expressed feeling, the sheer joy of being together, the pleasure of a free and uninhibited human interaction that kept alive the desire and the hope of our fathers. They also fought a great deal among themselves as Greeks somehow manage to do, but anger is feeling too, and it is an anger that emanates from that sense of individuality and personal dignity that perhaps is too readily violated. Here is the paradox of it all. The very traits that undergirded individual progress for Greeks also contributed to the slowing of their collective progress in America. Our fathers fought with their priests and bishops and presidents of their communities that they themselves had elected. They also found it difficult to engage in cooperative efforts with other Greeks in the business sphere of activities to combat the attacks of competitors. Organization was just not their "thing."

When a Greek was asked why he labored so hard, to what end were his efforts aimed, this response was consistent - - he was working for his children. It was in the generation that was to follow that the fullness of his desire and his hope were to be realized. His sons and his daughters would not work in the restaurant for long hours as he did. Theirs was to be a better and a fuller future. And so his "desire" and "hope" were transmitted to his children. It was reinforced in the afternoons in the Greek school of his

Church where he learned about the achievements of the ancient Greeks and the sacrifices of the modern Greeks who fought the enemies of their country. They were taught to be proud of their heritage, as their fathers were. They were imbued with the **potho** to live this heritage through their own individual achievements.

And the second generation fulfilled the dreams of their fathers. The sons and daughters of the original immigrants immersed themselves in their studies and entered a broad range of professions and businesses and distinguished themselves in this new country to which their fathers and their mothers had come. They progressed beyond their parents in a steady upward climb on the ladder of social mobility. Many climbed so long and reached so high that they could no longer see from where they had come. Or they did not care to. They were "Americans," they said; they had made it in American societal terms and they did not want to look back. They were embarassed now by the ways of the "old country" — those ways their parents had brought with them across the ocean. They also began to see the generation that had come before them to this country as swarthy men and women who spoke another one of those "peasant languages." They were embarrassed by the individual and collective "chauvinism" of their fathers and the "ethnocentrism" of the priests and bishops whom they encountered less and less. They were pained by the public displays of Greek nationalism on the twenty-fifth of March in the archaic insistence of the preservation of Greek culture in this country. They separated themselves as best they could from all of this. They also separated themselves from the source that had kindled and nurtured and preserved their desire and their hope to achieve; but they did not know this. They had also separated themselves from the community of caring - - that was the other gift their fathers had given to them. And they did not know this either. Their dedication to work and to individual achievement did not allow time for them to experience the loss of the sense of community that had sustained their fathers and their mothers. Greek celebrations on Easter Day and on those other special days of the year were a thing of the past, a thing of their childhoods. They did not miss the human experience of a joyful and spontaneous "being" together, that is the other half of the Greek way. They had taken another route, they told themselves; they had gone the "American" way.

In this trend, the Greek-Americans who were the children of the original immigrants were not different from their contemporaries who were the children of immigrants from other parts of Europe. They were all Americans, they told each other, of this or that national origin. They were Americans of Polish ancestry or Italian ancestry or Irish ancestry. They were all amalgamating into one huge melting pot that was to the America of the Future. Or so they thought.

In World War II, this commitment of American ethnic groups to their new country was sealed by the blood of their sons who fought alongside of "native" Americans - - that is, those who had come to this country before them - - on the battlefields of Europe and Asia. After the war the discrimination experienced by the more newly arrived immigrants in this country from those who had come before them lessened markedly. This country underwent then a period of unprecedented economic growth and members of ethnic groups were buoyed up by the new prosperity. They were able to obtain employment easily, salaries were good and the worker could even save enough to send his children to college. One's ethnic identity in these times was not held to open view. They were all Americans they told each other of this or that national origin. They did not like to be referred to as members of a sub-culture. There was a pejorative ring to this designation. They did not like to be called Italians or Poles or Greeks, the sons and daughters of immigrants. It was only during election periods that the ethnic composition of the populations of cities and states surfaced as an issue that needed to be taken into account by politicians who vied for public office. It was then that one heard of the Italo-American vote in the North End of Boston, or the Jewish vote in New York City. When the elections were over, references to ethnicity disappeared again from the American scene.

The burgeoning economy that characterized the post-war years in this country did not buoy up all the ethnics who had been woven into its social fabric. Black Americans could not share equally in the new prosperity and they were no longer content to sit by and watch themselves be left behind. Martin Luther King had a dream too. His dream was that Blacks and Whites would one day live together as equal partners in this new land to which his fathers had been brought long ago as slaves. They would share the prosperity of this rich land and live together as children of God. He was not to live to see his dream realized, and those of his brothers who came after him took a different direction from that which he had pointed out to them. The Black movement saw integration as a goal without hope of attainment. Militant Blacks turned away from that white society that had so long devalued them as less than human beings. Their rage erupted with a vengeance in Watts and in Newark and the decade of the sixties was shattered by riots in the cities and on the campuses of our country. When this rage had finally spent itself there were those among the Black leadership who said they could no longer live in this land that had for so long denied them the right to be men. They would return to the land which their fathers had been forced to leave as slaves and create a new society where they could live in dignity. Most Black Americans could not understand this. This was their country they said, and they had no intention of leaving it. They committed themselves instead to reaffirming their dignity as human beings in this country to which their fathers had been brought by white men as chattel on ships. "Black is beautiful" they declared and they served notice on white Americans that they would no longer be treated as second class citizens. Yes, they too had a culture which until now they had been reluctant to accept as their own. They knew they must rediscover their African heritage and identify with that far-away and strange land from which their fathers had been taken away in ships, as slaves. They knew that they needed a base on which to rebuild that sense of personal dignity that had been taken from them. Black consciousness was born in America.

Centers for the teaching of Black history and art were founded in Black neighborhoods, in high schools and on college campuses. Black culture now was nurtured as the common bond that revitalized the sense of Black consciousness and solidified the Black community into a force for change in this country. Before this, small numbers of Blacks were able to "make it" as individuals into white middle class society as professionals or businessmen. They, too, had felt their ethnicity to be a handicap in their efforts to be accepted by the White Anglo-Saxon Protestant majority. Now Blacks moved as a community to open the pathways to equal rights to economic opportunity for all their brethren. America listened now and a period of social and cultural change began that is still in progress.

The Black Movement spawned the Youth Movement. The youth of the nation who awakened to the injustices against Blacks saw that they were not limited to Blacks. They could now no longer tolerate the policies of their government which waged war against a people on the other side of the globe because they sought to determine their own political destiny. Protests against the Vietnam War disrupted our college campuses and our cities. The issue of freedom from discrimination became the rallying cry for other groups in this country. Mexican-American workers in the Southwest now found the injustices they had endured from their White Anglo-Saxon Protestant bosses intolerable and the Brown Movement was born. Indian-Americans whose cries for justice had been ignored for one hundred years as they lived huddled on their reservations now became vocal and assertive and the Red Movement was born. The rights of women to be treated as equals and not as the chattels of men were heralded by the Women's Liberation Movement.

When women protested they said that their dignity as human beings was being violated by men. When Mexican-Americans protested they said their dignity as an ethnic group was violated and so they reaffirmed their value as people separate from the White Anglo-Saxon Protestant society which surrounded them. The Indian-Americans shouted their rage at the characterization of their people as savages in movies and television and they too revitalized their sense of ethnic consciousness by reaffirming their cultural heritage.

But what about the White ethnics in all of this, those sons and daughters of immigrants from Italy and Poland and Ireland and Greece? At first they reacted with horror at the conflict that seemed to be engulfing their new country. They saw the Black Movement as an evil force and their sense of personal threat was heightened when Blacks moved into their neighborhoods or "invaded" their unions. Gradually, however, the vociferous determination by Blacks to be valued because of, rather than in spite of, the color of their skin earned the respect of White ethnics in whom a responsive chord had been struck. They could relate to this issue. Black ethnics had been forced to deny their cultural identity and their sense of personhood and were now actively reclaiming their right to be valued as a distinctive people. White ethnics had freely forfeited their cultural identities, which were their birthright, as Esau had forfeited his birthright - - for a bowl of economic properity - - and now they were ashamed. These sons and daughters of immigrants came forth slowly now also to reclaim what they had given away. An amazing thing began to happen in America. The melting pot had spilled over and it was discovered that very little amalgamation had taken place in this country among the different nationalities that were America. A study conducted in New York City in the early 1960's showed that the ethnic composition of that city had not changed much in a hundred years.[1] It remained, as it had always been, a Jewish, Puerto Rican and Black as well as Anglo-Saxon city. These ethnic groups, it was revealed, continued to maintain sub-cultures of their own in different parts of the city as they had always done. At the same time, the melting pot myth was perpetuated and was believed even by these ethnics themselves. The culturally heterogeneous configuration of America now began to show itself in progressively sharper stages of relief in the sixties.

Paradoxically, it was the children of the children of immigrants who assumed the leadership in this "new" trend to reaffirm openly their traditional cultural roots. It was the third generation ethnics,

---

[1] See Nathan Glazer and Daniel P. Moynihan's Beyond the Melting Pot (Cambridge: MIT Press, 1963).

those grandchildren of the original immigrants who came forth to rekindle the sense of ethnic consciousness that their fathers and their mothers, the sons and daughters of immigrants, had rejected. How could this be? What motivated this third generation of ethnic Americans to seek out and to reaffirm their cultural heritages? They held well-paying jobs in working class occupations and increasingly large numbers of them were entering the professions where their economic and social positions were being secured in the social structure.

They came forth because they shared with all of America's youth a sense of personal isolation and anomie in their own country. The discrepancy in America between the overt professed values of equality and democracy and the now apparent institutionalization of discrimination such as that against Blacks, against Mexican-Americans, against American Indians, and against women left them disillusioned and angry. But that was only the half of it. The other half of their dissatisfaction emanated from the quality of life itself in this country. Third generation ethnic Americans shared with the sons and daughters of "native" Americans a dissatisfaction with those middle class core values that are the life experience in the United States. The Protestant work ethic with its primary emphasis on individual achievement at the price of other human values was now being questioned by many of America's youth. Was life to be lived solely for individual material gain, where competition characterized the relationship between men and women and where one's individual worth as a human being was judged wholly on how far he or she had climbed up the ladder of economic success? Were human relationships to be valued solely on the degree to which they were instrumental in enhancing this continuing drive to upward social mobility? What about the joy of human relationships experienced for what they are rather than for what they will get us, of caring for one another, of working with each other toward the attainment of common human goals that supersede our individual material interests? Where were these human needs for "mutuality," as Erickson labeled them, to be satisfied?[2] Was this emotional sterility, this "pursuit of loneliness" that is the natural by-product of unbridled competitive striving to be the reward of "making it" in the "system."[3] Many of America's youth, among them the most

---

[2]See Erik H. Erickson's Childhood and Society (New York: Norton Press, 1950).

[3]See Philip Slater's The Pursuit of Loneliness: American Culture at the Breaking Point (Boston: Beacon Press, 1970).

privileged, chose to reject the "system" in the 1960's. They took a variety of routes. The drug sub-culture created a crisis in America. The more radical among the youth formed groups to oppose the war in Vietnam, others established communes where they experimented with alternate, i.e., non-middle class life styles. America's youth who were the grandchildren of immigrants chose to reaffirm their ethnic identities. They remembered a different life when they were growing up and it made their current feelings of isolation and anomie even harder to bear.

The open manifestation of ethnic feelings took a variety of forms, and also varied in intensity, in different White sub-cultural groups. In New York City, the Italian-American Fraternal Society organized itself to combat the prejudicial stereotyping of Italian gangsters in movie and television films. Its program was also positively geared to affirming the contributions made by the Italian-Americans to American society. Polish-American cultural and fraternal organizations also took more aggressive stands against the mass media for stereotyping their ethnic group. Pulaski Day in the sixties drew an unprecedented number of second and third generation Polish-Americans who in previous years had left the celebration of the memory of that World War I Polish-American war hero to their fathers and grandfathers. Greek-Americans organized themselves into a national organization named the Greek Orthodox of America (G.O.Y.A.). It is important to note that the primary impetus for this effort of Greek Americans did not come from the fraternal and cultural organizations founded earlier by their immigrant fathers and grandfathers. Nor did it come from the Greek Orthodox Church. It came from the second and third generation youths themselves who felt the need to unite for the purpose of deepening their sense of Greek consciousness.

Perhaps the most dramatic manifestation of this reaffirmation of ethnic origins was the response of young American Jews to Israeli-Arab conflicts - - first in 1967 and then in 1973. The war in 1967 stirred a deep interest in thousands of young American Jews. The Israeli victory after only six days of fighting was experienced by them as a personal triumph. Many followed up their emotional involvement in this conflict by going to Israel and working on kibbutzim and in other settings with the clear purpose of making a contribution to Israel. They believed that in the process they were also renewing themselves. It felt right to commit themselves to a cause outside the realm of their individual social and economic advancement. It satisfied the need for the "mutuality" that Erickson had taught them was an essential ingredient of a healty personality. When the Israeli-Arab conflict was activated again in 1973, the response of American Jews was overwhelming. Young men and women left their schools and jobs and professions and traveled to Israel to participate in whatever way they could.

This open affirmation of ethnic identity signals a new period in the social and cultural evolution of America. There is a "new pluralism" developing in this country which promises to restructure the relationship of minority groups to the dominant Anglo-Saxon Protestant White culture. This "new pluralism" will provide a system of relationships which accepts the uniqueness of sub-cultural groups and balances their ethnic identification with commitment to American society as a whole.[4]

The choices faced by the second generation of ethnic Americans in the past of either identifying with their subcultures and isolating themselves from the mainstream of American society, or becoming completely "Americanized" and so rejecting an important part of themselves are no longer the only viable ones in this country. It has now become clear that another alternative has developed as a consequence of the events of the 1960's. This alternative is based on the open recognition that ethnic variation is and always has been an integral part of the American scene. It is now possible for members of ethnic groups openly to identify with their cultural heritage while committing themselves to an American sense of national purpose. In fact the very process that is now making it possible for members of ethnic groups to feel free to assert their individual and collective uniqueness within the broader social system is also awakening within them a common sense of American consciousness. Individually and collectively we can be strengthened psychologically and socially as we move freely between our sub-cultures where we are renewed by our cultural roots that reach back to the old world and which provide us with resources for achievement and growth in the new world. We are at the beginning in this country of this effort to create the "new pluralism" that is to be the America of the future.

I would like finally to share with you some of my thoughts on the implication of this "new pluralism" for Greeks in America. Our fathers we can see now - - those originals Greeks like my old friend who came to this country as a boy - - granted us a legacy that we are only now coming fully to appreciate. For the second

---

[4]The American Jewish Committee, "Pluralism beyond the Frontier," Report of the San Francisco Consultation on Ethnicity (San Francisco: The American Jewish Committee, 1971).

generation, Greek culture provided a source of motivation to achieve in a country where survival itself is dependent on achievement. For the third generation, it can provide the cultural basis for individual identification and the enhancement of the sense of personhood in a period marked by alienation and anomie. It need no longer separate Greek Americans from other Americans, neither from "native" Americans nor from other ethnic Americans of this or that national origin. It can keep alive the **potho**, the "desire" and the "hope" for a better tomorrow in a strong and a free America, and it can teach us how to "care for one another."

CRISIS IN MARRIAGE AND THE FAMILY

PSYCHOLOGICAL PERSPECTIVE

by Diane Coulopoulos

Everyone is acutely aware of the crisis in marriage and the family. A review of the literature or even daily reading of the newspaper bombards us with the most recent frightening statistics on the subject. For example, one in every three marriages ends in divorce; more than half of the nation's 59.1 million children have working mothers; and up to 50% of the children will at some time live in a single-parent family (Boston Globe, November 1981). It is interesting to note that Massachusetts has a higher percentage of single parents and working mothers than the nation as a whole.

Additional data indicate that 40% of all married adults will get divorced at least once. In the United States, nearly 25% of all children are presently living with one parent who is divorced or separated or with a parent who has remarried after divorce.[1]

---

[1] M. K. Montieth, "The Reading Teacher vs Children of Divorce," The Reading Teacher (Volume 35, Number 1), October, 1981.

Dr. Diane Coulopoulos has been Professor of Psychology at Simmons College since 1965. She is also Project Director of a federally funded program, Project TEAM, "Training for Equal Assessment for Minorities." She has worked as a consultant to St. Basil's Academy in Garrison, New York, and also to the public schools. She has recently published Self Concept and Education: A Guide for Teachers and Parents, Athens, Greece: Alkyond Press, 1982.

How is the Greek Orthodox marriage or family reflected in these figures? An examination of the vital statistics for the decade, 1970-1980, provided by the Greek Orthodox Archdiocese gives us some information. The data includes figures on the number of weddings, baptisms, funerals and divorces recorded in the Greek Archdiocese for North and South America between the years 1970-1979. In a six year period (1970-1976) there were 3,227 divorces; in a three year period (1977-1979) there were 1,896 divorces, which indicates an acceleration in the number of divorces. It should also be noted that during those last three years, there were actually fewer marriages. Another important set of data are the figures on the Greek Orthodox as compared to the mixed marriages (Greek Orthodox and non Greek Orthodox) and divorces. The number of Greek Orthodox and mixed marriages are very similar. In contrast, however, the divorce rate for Greek Orthodox couples is much higher than that of the mixed marriage couples[2] (See Table 1).

TABLE 1

	1976	1977	1978
Greek Orthodox Marriages	2,537	2,521	2,295
Mixed Marriages	2,201	2,438	2,445
Greek Orthodox Divorce	350	358	419
Mixed Divorce	201	223	256

One must be cautious in making inferences based on these data. It is safe to say that there are a large number of children who are affected by divorce in the Archdiocese. It should also be pointed out that there are no data on separated parents, homes with only one parent due to the death of a spouse or unwed parents.

These data also raise interesting questions with respect to the stability of marriages in our Church and the factors that contribute to the success or failures of Greek Orthodox marriages. Is the instability of Greek Orthodox marriages due to immaturity and prolonged dependence of young Greek adults? Does the Greek family have expectations that conflict with those of the majority culture? Are Greek men unable to deal with the changing roles and expectations of Greek women?

Another factor to examine is the working mother. Economic factors

[2]Vital Statistics of the Greek Orthodox Archdiocese of North and South America, 1970-1980 (New York, New York: Greek Orthodox Archdiocese).

today, as well as increased materialism, have resulted in a change in the family structure. This is especially important to the recent immigrant, who faces not only the stresses of entering a new culture, but finds that he or she must also deal with the changing nature and function of the family; one of those changes, for example, is the mother who immediately enters the workforce.

Since in most divorces there are children involved, I would like to address the impact of the divorce on the family system. Families experience a great deal of stress and change which are directly related to the alteration in parent-child interaction. While we consider the model of the nuclear family unit to be composed of husband, wife and children, only 44% of families in the United States correspond to this model.[3]

In most divorces involving children, the mother still receives custody of the child although there has been an increase in the proportion of children living with their fathers. It is important to consider here how the change in the family structure, with the resulting stress and coping strategies, are related to the parent-child relation. A number of practical problems are encountered by divorced parents, such as household maintenance, and economic and occupational difficulties. One of the consequences of divorce is the reported "chaotic life style" which includes problems in dealing with routine household chores and maintaining an ordered and scheduled life (eating meals together, going to bed at a regular time, being on time for school, etc.). This is particularly the case during the first year after divorce but tends to improve over time.[4]

It has been found that during the first year following divorce, divorced mothers and fathers feel more anxious, depressed, angry, rejected and incompetent. Interestingly, divorced mothers of sons feel less competent, more anxious, more angry and more externally controlled as measured by the I-E Scale, than do married mothers and divorced mothers of girls.[5] This is important in light of the evidence that the mother-son relationship is especially problematic

---

[3] R. and R. N. Rapaport and Z. Stulitz, Fathers, Mothers and Society: Perspectives on Parenting (New York, New York: Vintage Books, 1980).

[4] Hetherington and M. and R. Cox, "The Aftermath of Divorce," in Contemporary Readings in Child Psychology (New York, New York: McGraw Hill, 1981).

[5] Ibid.

in divorced families.

It is apparent that the divorced parents undergo a great deal of difficulty and stress: for some fathers, there is a strong sense of loss; for both husbands and wives, there is a decline in self esteem and competence.

Returning to the parent-child interaction, during the first several months after divorce, fathers tend to have high contact with their children. In time, however, this pattern changes, and by the end of two years the contact is dramatically reduced.

Poor parenting is noted with the divorced parent as compared to non-divorced parents in terms of: 1. fewer maturity demands made upon their children; 2. less communication with their children; 3. less expressed affection; 4. marked inconsistency in discipline; and 5. lack of control over their children. The data indicate that divorced parents communicate less, are less consistent, and use more negative sanctions with their sons than with their daughters. Mothers have the greatest problems in interacting with their sons. It seems that sons of divorced parents "have a hard time of it" and, consequently, the adverse affects of divorce are more severe and enduring for boys than for girls.

In a study of Hetherington[6] it was found that children of divorced parents exhibit more negative behavior than children of intact families. These behaviors are also more marked in boys than girls and have dissipated in girls by the end of two years after divorce. Children of divorce also exhibit more negative behavior in the presence of their mothers than their fathers. There appears to be a pattern which indicates that boys are more oppositional and aggressive than girls toward their mothers and that girls are more whining, complaining, and compliant. These children nag, complain and make more dependency demands, and are more likely to ignore their mothers.

It is fair to ask who is doing what to whom in this situation. It seems that mothers and their aggressive children get caught up in a vicious cycle of coercion. These mothers tend to have poor management skills which accelerates the child's aversive behavior for which she is the main instigator and target. The mother reacts by increasing coercion in her parenting behavior with accompanying

---

[6] Ibid.

feelings of helplessness, depression, anger and self-doubt.[7] In his research, Patterson found that mothers who received treatment aimed at improving parenting skills showed improvement on a number of clinical scales on the MMPI, as well as a decrease in the noxious behaviors of their aggressive children.

Another interesting finding is that fathers tended to be less affected by a problem child than were mothers.[8] This can be attributed to three factors: 1. fathers spend less time with their children; 2. children exhibit less deviant behavior in the presence of their fathers; and 3. fathers can control deviant behavior better when it does occur.

Support in child rearing from the spouse and agreement with the spouse in disciplining the child in both divorced and intact families is effective in dealing with the child. We find a positive mother-child interaction and a more positive adjustment of the child when the following conditions exist: 1. agreement in child rearing; 2. a positive attitude toward the spouse; 3. low conflict between the divorced parents; 4. the father is emotionally mature; and 5. there is frequent contact between father and child. When these conditions are absent, and there is conflict, ill will and emotional immaturity in the father and the mother, the consequences are predictably bad.

Support systems are found to be related to a mother's effectiveness in coping and interacting with her child. Such systems include grandparents, siblings, close friends (especially other divorced friends) or competent housekeeper or male friends with whom there is an intimate relationship. For the father, women with whom he is intimately involved, married friends and relatives result in the next greatest support in his relationship with his children.

These children of divorce do suffer from the stress which is expressed in anger, guilt, feelings of loneliness and isolation. These feelings do affect the child's ability to perform well in the classroom and affect accompanying behaviors such as moodiness, withdrawal, declining grades and acting out.

---

[7] Patterson, G. "Mothers: The Unacknowledged Victims." Paper presented at the Western Regional Meetings for the Society for Research in Child Development, (Oakland, California: April 1976).

[8] Ibid.

Divorce is one of the most serious crises in contemporary American life. The need to develop support systems is critical to help parents cope with the changes that occur because of divorce. Support systems are needed to prevent or to modify the harmful consequences that accompany the disruption of the traditional family unit. The mental health profession and the church can play an important role here. One way is by providing treatment or services that relate directly to effective parenting; such services can furnish concrete methods of dealing with immediate parent-child interaction and assist the parent in dealing with his or her sense or competency and self-esteem.

CRISIS IN MARRIAGE AND THE FAMILY

THEOLOGICAL PERSPECTIVE

by Arthur Metaxas

The family unit is being challenged by many forces which, in time, may make it become an endangered species. But at least endangered species down to the smallest fish, bird or animal are protected by the federal government from possible extinction while millions of dollars in humanitarian projects are curtailed. Who is going to protect the sanctity of the family and how much is it going to cost in lives and human suffering before some resolute and definitive action is taken by responsible authorities? What can we do about it?

The family is under attack from many sides. The liberals have had their day and their say. It is time for the rest of us to stand up and be heard in a most convincing manner. Family relationships have reached a low ebb. The evolvement of single parent homes poses a great threat to the institution of the family upon which the stability and solidarity of society depends.

The Reverend Fr. Arthur J. Metaxas is Pastor of St. Athanasios the Great Greek Orthodox Church in Arlington, Massachusetts. He serves as Chaplain to the AHEPA and to the Minutemen in Lexington, Massachusetts. Fr. Metaxas also provides counseling services to adolescents and to family members of the parish.

As in other cultures, the Greek cultural roots in the past, and to a great extent even today, have contributed to unity, harmony and balance in the Greek home. The retention of certain cultural traditions and customs has been partially responsible for maintaining a sense of identity, a sense of belonging, a sense of allegiance to the family and a sense of determination in keeping the family spirit alive.

One sociologist who has studied the rituals of hundreds of families, points out that families with the strongest ties have the most rituals: "They are important not so much for whatever is said and done," he says, "but for the results they yield - - the sense of 'we-ness' that grows out of shared experience, and the feeling of 'rightness' that comes from its repetitions. More than anything, the ritual is a symbol of how family members feel about one another."

Most rituals, of course, crystallize around traditional occasions. At Christmas, for example, many families have special ways of exchanging gifts. Thanksgiving and birthday rituals usually center around food. At one time, for the Greek Orthodox Christians, the celebration of a feast day was more important than that of a birthday. It was associated with a religious and saintly person. Church attendance was crucial to this observance. Relatives and friends were invited to the home to celebrate the feast day. Unfortunately, this enviable practice has now become virtually extinct because we have become too involved with other mundane concerns.

Family rituals, however, are just as likely to grow out of spontaneous or chance events as they are of more established traditions rooted in the past. One woman unwittingly started a ritual when she and her husband were taking an inventory of their household possessions for a fire insurance policy. When the job was finished she said, "Well, we know what **things** we have, but what about the intangibles? So we made another list of qualities like love, trust, good health, a sense of humour - - what we call our happiness inventory. Now, once a year we review it and try to add an item or two to the list."

Most families, however, are guilty of subtracting or not adding anything to the happiness inventory. Rather, they keep on adding items to their material inventory.

Why are family rituals important? What basic purposes do they serve?

They Reinforce Family Closeness.

Says a woman whose busy family is rarely at home at dinner time, "There is always a candle in the centerpiece of the table, but I light it only when we are all there at the same time. When it goes unlighted for many days in a row, we all make a special effort to be home."

How often do we gather to eat together as a family? How much time do we spend at the dinner table discussing mutual problems and concerns? Very little I'm afraid. Our candle then remains unlit for a long, long time.

Rituals Enhance a Family's Sense of Stability and Emotional Security.

For young children, bedtime rituals are a source of comfort and reassurance. It's unfortunate when only the baby sitter is present to put the child to be.

Rituals put a Special Stamp on Family Milestones.

One man remembers being taken on a hunting trip with his father when he turned sixteen years of age: "It was the first time just the two of us went into the woods, and I knew it was his way of saying that I was grown up. I've done the same thing with my own sons."

Thus, if wisely cultivated, rituals provide the sense of continuity, understanding and love that strengthens family closeness. As one woman puts it, "Rituals are family keepsakes that live in your heart."

How many of us take time out to do things with our children? We are always on the go. We have so many commitments and appointments to keep. However for us there are no traffic lights. We do not proceed with caution so as to avoid any impending danger. We do not stop on red to ascertain if the road is clear ahead before we proceed. We do not stop to reassess our journey in life and take corrective steps to change our course and our direction. All we see is the green light which encourages us to step on the accelerator and to keep on going at a faster and faster rate of speed without any thought of detours and obstacles on the road ahead.

Undeniably, certain pressures, tensions and tendencies have contributed greatly to the steady disintegration of the family unit with predictable results. The idealistic assumption of eternal love and devotion has suffered tragically. It has been undermined by so many negative factors. We may be victims of the romantic illusion that love is something which happens to you at first sight, and there is nothing you can do about it. Is this why hopes are often unachieved and the divorce rate is climbing to a point where one out of every three marriages ends in divorce?

Is it due to the fact that more than half of the children in the U. S. have mothers who work away from home as part of the civilian labor force, as indicated by a recent Labor Department report? In 1980, 52.8 percent of American children had working mothers, while in 1970, only 38.9 percent were in that category.

Is it because one out of every six families is maintained by a woman who is either divorced, separated, widowed or never married?

Is it because of changing times and changing pressures that our youngsters, exposed to erotic stimuli, succumb and become involved, attempting in the process to find fulfillment, to satisfy a supposedly deeper need?

Is it because many parents use alcohol with the tragic result that our youth accept this behavior as the norm and are, therefore, easily led into drugs? Three million youngsters, some as young as 11 and 12 years old, have become addicted to alcohol. We have progressed tremendously from an intellectual standpoint but we have failed dismally from a spiritual standpoint.

Is it because 33% of the housewives in this country have become addicted to alcohol, making it impossible for them to fulfill their roles, and as a result, the entire family suffers? What are their needs which are not being met?

Is it because 200,000 children are physically abused by parents and guardians and that the number of battered wives is increasing at an alarming rate?

Years ago, in times of need and distress, the members of the clergy were the first to be contacted for support, compassion and understanding. Today, this tendency is not as evident because the Church has been stereotyped as an institution with entrenched, rigid, unyielding moral values - - an institution that has many untrained clergymen who are unable to cope with the complexities or modern life. Consequently, many of our disturbed and distressed faithful turn to psychologists and psychiatrists, who are not religiously oriented, and to various cults in an attempt to achieve that elusive end - - an integrated liberated personality.

At this point in our discussion, it is incumbent upon us to present some ideas designed to facilitate a more positive and healty impact on our faithful. The church, in her role as builder of family life, will continue as an effective institution only as she is supported by happy, stable and spiritually health families. Hence, pre-marital counseling is of tremendous importance to the church. The primary need is to inaugurate a definite premarital counseling program and erase, to an appreciable degree, the somewhat disgraceful practice of marrying persons who do not have the slightest knowledge of what the relationship entails.

For those already married, marriage counseling can be a valuable tool. Essentially, marriage counseling is no different than any other kind of counseling. What is being called "marriage" counseling centers on problems arising in marriage. The help which is needed is in the area of inner attitudes, feelings and needs. The persons involved need help to face, to understand and to give up childish and immature feelings and responses, and to achieve a more mature kind of relationship within the marriage situation.

Theological education in the past has been grossly deficient in the area of counseling. We were sent out into the arena of public life without the necessary tools to deal effectively with the emotional and psychological problems which beset our faithful. That meant we had to go it alone. Today the situation is quite different. Today our students are receiving field education and are taking courses in pastoral psychology which prepare them to deal more adequately with spiritual and psychological problems. This advancement in educational training means that the theological school accepts a much greater responsibility for the growth of the student as a person.

One of the most useful and beneficial means of preparing the student to be an effective counselor is not only to provide courses in counseling theory but also to provide actual counseling opportunities under supervision. This is where a great many errors in judgment can be corrected, a deeper understanding of problems can be achieved and theological misconceptions can be resolved. For the pastor who would help others must first be helped to grow himself, through both the counseling and the learning processes.

The pastor must be sensitive to the needs of individuals. He must be adept in meeting those needs. He must utilize the resources which his Faith has to offer, because for those of us from a Christian background, if marriages are not made in heaven they will never make it here on earth. For it is truly written, "Except the Lord build the house, they labor in vain who build it." The love of God, the forgiveness of God and the reconciliation with God can be invaluable in alleviating the pain of anxiety and guilt. It is unfortunate that it is extremely difficult for man to offer love, forgiveness and reconciliation to his fellow man.

The ministry of the Church, however, is not restricted only to those contemplating marriage and to those who are already married. The Church has an obligation to meet effectively the problems confronting the youth, the widowed, the divorced, the separated, the single individual, the senior citizen, the children of divorced or separated parents, the alcoholic, the handicapped and the underprivileged. This suggests that the pastor is expected to be all things to all people - - clearly an impossible task. The sensitive pastor can only offer help to the limits of his expertise. Beyond that he must have the intuitive grasp to comprehend which concerns are beyond his comprehension. This means that he must know when and to whom to refer the individual for further counseling without feeling that he has failed. Even after referral, the pastor should stay in touch with the counselee; to be a continuing resource, to demonstrate the Church's great concern for his or her welfare, and to stress the Church's role as a builder of spiritual health in individuals as well as families.

ADOLESCENCE: CONFLICTS AND IDENTITY

PSYCHOLOGICAL PERSPECTIVE

by Maximi Anastos

Editor's Note: Dr. Anastos spoke extemporaneously from brief notes which are presented here. Her talk was based on case discussions which demonstrated the points of her presentation.

ADOLESCENCE

Adolescence is the state or period of growth from puberty to maturity. Its beginning is marked by the appearance of secondary sexual characteristics at about age 12; its termination is at about age 20. In this period sexual maturity is achieved. It is the age of final establishment of a dominant positive ego identity in which the ego must achieve independence: the old emotional ties must be cast off and new attachments made.

Biological development brings great qualitative and quantitative changes in both the physiological and psychological areas. The ego is confronted with new difficulties and conflicts. Because these changes are closely connected with instinctual life, the emotions

---

Dr. Maximi Anastos is Chief Psychiatrist at Beaverbrook Guidance Center in Watertown, Massachusetts. She is Staff Psychiatrist at Mt. Auburn Hospital, Cambridge, Massachusetts and a Psychiatric Consultant at the Social Security Disability Determination Office in Boston. She also maintains a private practice in psychotherapy in Cambridge.

are affected more than any other part of the personality.

Young people can become remarkably intolerant and cruel in their exclusion of others who are "different" in cultural background, in tastes, in dress, etc. They develop "cliques." Such intolerance may be, for a while, a necessary defense against a sense of identity loss when the immediate future presents too many conflicting possibilities and choices. Relying to a great extent on the peer group, young people not only help each other by sharing their feelings, their ideals and even their enemies, but they also test each other's capacity for loyalties and values.

The quiet behavior of the "Latency Period," when the child has been behaving "well" - - i.e., obedient, responsible, confident, etc., will often be replaced by opposite behavior during the adolescent period. The impression of health and rationality disappears. The pre-adolescent seems to be less mature, less "normal," selfish and inconsiderate. In more severe cases, he or she may behave anti-socially or even somewhat psychotically. The pre-adolescent may express idealism and/or altruism or may respond critically. Generally, this pathology disappears when adolescence has run its course.

This stressful situation is called "Developmental Conflicts." The adolescents wake up from the comforting dependency on their parents who so far have been making the decisions for them. They realize that from now on they have to be independent. This is a very scary and anxiety-provoking realization. How will they make all these decisions? How will they find out what they like? (A fifteen year old girl told me, "I am confused. I don't know what I like. How do I know what I like is best for me? Everybody at home treats me like a baby. No one gives me the impression that I know anything.")

Introspection (looking into oneself) in adolescence can be a mental pain. It is only through identification with a successful and trusted adult with whom the adolescent is in alliance and whom he or she idealizes that the adolescent will be able to overcome these developmental conflicts and become a successful adult himself or herself. Thus, adults have a big responsibility to help adolescents by projecting a successful image in their adult role.

HOW TO HELP ADOLESCENTS

Being with or living with an adolescent can be an exciting and interesting experience or a very frustrating experience. Parents should be prepared and anticipate. They should not get "panicky" when they see their "good child" behaving in a way they do not approve (A father got panicky when his 16 year old son asked for permission to take a girl classmate to a movie. He started having the most destructive fantasies about his son's future: that he would drop out of school; that he would not go on to college; that he would get married and be unable to support his family, etc. The father's history, on the other hand, showed that he had started dating at 13. My response to him was that he should be grateful that his son is healthy and that he is growing up).

What adolescents need from adults is understanding, comforting, privacy, flexibility, fair and consistent rules and discipline, education and help in understanding themselves. They need to know that it takes time to learn how to become an adult.

Above all, adults, and parents in particular, should trust adolescents. Basically they know what is right and what is wrong. The message which give them strength is that we trust them not to something for which they will feel shame for themselves or for their family.

ADOLESCENTS: CONFLICTS AND IDENTITY

THEOLOGICAL PERSPECTIVE

by Nick A. Milas

"When the rulers are at peace who is there to divide and break up this peace? On the other hand, when they do not find themselves on good terms, nothing will be healthy in the household."[1] So writes St. John Chrysostom to Titus as he explains the effects of parental development on children's growth. With his words in mind, we can imagine the plight of the adolescent as he/she enters the end of this twentieth century. Adolescents characteristically question the values of society if only to be reassured that some stability does exist outside of them. But look at the obstacles an adolescent must face today.

---

[1] St. John Chrysostom, "Homilies on the Epistles of St. Paul the Apostle to Timothy, Titus, and Philemon," Nicene and Post-Nicene Fathers of the Christian Church, Vol. XIII, ed. Philip Schaff (Grand Rapids, Michigan: Wm. B. Eerdmans Publishing Co., 1979), p. 24.

Reverend Nick A. Milas is Pastor of "The Assumption" Greek Orthodox Church in Pawtucket, Rhode Island. He is Orthodox Chaplain at the Veteran's Soldier's Home in Bristol and Women and Infants Hospital in Providence. He also serves on the New England Greek Orthodox Diocesan Youth Commission.

Just using the topics of today's symposium as a point of reference, we can see that he/she is dealing with a society which reinforces adolescent behavior rather than a society which helps him/her grow out of it. Where in school are there supports and reinforcers for his/her identity as an Orthodox Christian or as a Greek? Where on television, or in the music he/she hears, are values espoused which offer him/her some direction in what he/she often perceives as a chaotic, cruel and unfair world? If father is facing a mid-life crisis or losing his job and most of his self-esteem, who will reflect for the adolescent the virtues of wisdom and foresight?[2] If mother is seeking personal fulfillment or enrichment of some sort - - or barely able to cope at all with middle age, faces economic strain or a husband ready to desert her where will the adolescent find motherly compassion?[3] If marriages fail even before they begin and the family core has been relegated to the family bore, then how can those members of our community who are in such a state of turmoil have their needs met? They will and they do, in fact, turn to each other, to the peer group - - and that is where they find outlets in sex and drugs and learn to express their frustration and anger in many negative and self-destructive ways.

When Fritz Redl began his work with delinquent youths, he identified many of the characteristics of adolescence which we understand today as adolescent behavior.[4] While constructing a therapeutic intervention for troubled and delinquent adolescents, he found that structure is absolutely necessary. His work led him to the conclusion that routine, rituals and regulations are indispensable. They make for predictability. They give order to an otherwise disorderly world. It is this need for routine, ritual and regulation that the Orthodox Church meets. Orthodoxy as a therapeutic intervention for adolescents has no modern rival. There is no one system, approach or orientation which can compare to the wide scope of effectiveness of the Church.

Let us look at just a few of the ways that the Orthodox Church can help the adolescent:

---

[2] John K. Campbell, Honour, Family and Patronage: A Study of Institutions and Moral Values in a Greek Mountain Community (Oxford: Clarendon Press, Inc., 1964), p. 37.

[3] Ibid.

[4] Fritz Redl, Our Troubles with Defiant Youth (London, England: The Free Press, Inc., 1957).

The first observable symptom of adolescence is rebellion. Particularly rebellion against parents. Parents themselves react in many ways. Often they feel, "How could my child act this way?" Sometimes they are self-deprecating: "Where did I go wrong?" Sometimes they try to minimize the situation by explaining it away - - "It's just a stage he's going through." The intervention, the remedy, the therapy is a two-sided coin. On the one side are the parents. Church workers can help those parents by knowing and recognizing what is going on. We can offer support and comfort to them. We can say, "You are not alone. I/we have gone through this or are going through this." We can give them a chance to let off steam, express some negative feelings or just give them a shoulder to lean on.

One might ask, who are the church workers? They are many people: the priest, seminarians, church school teachers, language teachers, choir member, chanters, custodial help, trustees and Philoptochos members, the people who Sunday after Sunday, year after year, seem to be posted at their respective stations. They are publicly visible and the communicants know who they are. Hearing empathetic words from community leaders such as these can be extremely helpful and comforting.[5]

The other side of the coin is to consider the struggle of the adolescent. He or she is seeking to find an identity. In order to do so he/she must separate from the parents. The more painful the separation the noisier the rebellion. But he/she cannot be without parents. With all those church workers around him/her the adolescent can very often find a parent figure or model with whom he/she can relate and with whom he/she can identify. We have already begun doing this more existentially in our catechistic programs. A new emphasis has been placed on learning about the lives of saints. Our young people are hungry for it. The paradigm is not new but it cannot be stated enough. For all of us, but particularly for the adolescent, God and the priest become fathers and the Theotokos and the Church become comforters and nurturers. In many cases, the young person will rebel and express his anger, but if the church workers know and expect this response, it will not be shocking or upsetting to them. Consistent and predictable response to an adolescent goes a long way. This does not mean a "poor you" attitude. Rather, it reflects the understanding that

---

[5] Richard Almond, <u>The Healing Community: Dynamics of the Therapeutic Milieu</u> (New York, New York: Jason Anderson, Inc., 1974), p. 311.

all mankind is struggling, that everyone is a sinner, and that our experience can be openly shared.

One of many stories of the desert fathers talks about this sharing. A young man was "harrassed by the demon of lust." He went to one old man who condemned him for his feelings. So, he decided to leave the community - - just as so many adolescents do who, after perceiving they have failed, drop out of the family, the school, and the Church.[6] As he was leaving, he encountered the Abbott Apollo, who asked him about his sad demeanor. The young man described his inner conflict to the Abbott, who confessed that even at his old age, after many years of the ascetic life, he too was harrassed by many temptations. Upon hearing that, the young man felt better and decided to remain in the community.[7]

Another plague of adolescence is low self-esteem or generalized insecurity about the self. Adolescents need feedback, although they find positive feedback embarrasing and negative feedback humiliating. Here is where the role of the Church can be helpful. The sacrament of Confession is indispensible for adolescents. It is a place for them to talk about themselves without fear of public humiliation. It is a place where they can be private and close the door and still not be alone. The priest in Confession represents many people to that young person. He is God's representative telling an adolescent who feels badly about himself, "I think you are okay." He is a friend who can hear all the secrets but will not tell, no matter what. He is a parent, an authority figure, who does not pose any threat to that individual's autonomy. The priest represents the Church in confession and as Lossky tells us, "The Church is the center of the universe, the sphere in which its destinies are determined. All are called to enter into the Church, for if Man is a microcosm, the Church is a macro-anthropos. It increases and is compounded in history, bringing the elect into its bosom and uniting them to God."[8] So the adolescent who in the family and in school feels continuously challenged to assert his/her

---

[6] Vernon Jones, Adolescents with Behavioral Problems: Strategies for Teaching, Counseling, and Parent Involvement (New York: Allyn, Inc., 1979).

[7] Helen Waddell, trans., The Desert Fathers (Ann Arbor, Mihigan: The University of Michigan Press., Inc., 1966), pp. 74-75.

[8] Vladimir Lossky, The Mystical Theology of the Eastern Church (London, England: James Clark and Company, Ltd., 1957), p. 178.

autonomy can have it verified by the entire Church, for at least that short time in Confession.

Adolescence is also a time for pendulum emotions. One day he/she is feeling like the master of the universe - - Luke Skywalker having overcome the black force for all time. The next day he/she is plunged into the depths of depression and has yet to hit the bottom. Routine, ritual and regulations are needed, Redl tells us. The liturgical life of the Orthodox Church is limited only by our own ability to participate. The Divine Services express many highs and lows. They talk about enemies and God's love, man's sins and God's mercy. While attending, the adolescent gets to satisfy that one, constant nagging wish - - to get out of the house. He/she also uses that energy which sometimes is so abundant. And when depression and exhaustion invariably ensue, he/she can lean over a book, or just look at all the visual reminders of God's love and Incarnation (that is of course, icons) which are a lesson and a comfort in themselves.

What about the adolescent's need for routine? This need may be satisfied easily enough by fasting. Fasting can be his own private way of participating in the life of the Church. As a way of instituting routine, fasting can have many positive side effects. First, it makes the adolescent aware of the passing of time. First Wednesday, then Friday, then Sunday, then it is time to fast for Christmas and Great Lent and the Holy Apostles and the fast of Dormition. Always some celebration lies ahead. Always some indication that time is not standing still but really is passing and the hope exists that his/her personal struggle and suffering will effect closure of some sort.

Then there is the concept of cleansing. Adolescents are often guilt ridden about their behavior, their anger or their sense of inadequacy because they perceive that they are failing their parents, teachers, and other significant adults. Fasting helps draw them away from their self-centeredness. Knowing how concerned they are about physical attractiveness and the opposite sex, fasting gives them a constructive way of focusing on their bodies without guilt. They can begin at this point in their life cycle to understand that their bodies are not only a means of deriving pleasure and gratification, but also a vehicle to salvation - - a way of finding the Kingdom and learning that the body is a potential vessel of God's Grace.

And, finally there is prayer. Those of us who have adolescents in our home know how much time they spend behind closed doors.

One wonders what he/she can be doing for so many hours. The bottom line is, he/she is trying to fill the void. He/she is trying to find out "what's wrong with me" or trying to prove "I'm okay." There are so many avenues the adolescent can pursue in terms of prayer and meditation. There is the simple Jesus Prayer, which can be used according to the guidelines of the Confessor or according to one of the books on this subject available today (Ware's "The Power of the Name," Brianchaninov's "On the Prayer of Jesus," and Bloom's "Beginning to Pray" are some of the more popular and easy to read). There are pocket prayer books, with a variety of prayers ranging from forgiveness to thanksgiving. There are spiritual writings, lives of saints, the Gospel and the entire Bible, of course. All these the adolescent can take into his/her private place. And more importantly, he/she can bring them out as well, and grow in the use of them as he/she grows emotionally and spiritually.

I suspect that there are parents, teachers, church workers and even clergy who will contend that community support, Confession, Divine Services, fasting and prayer are not the route to go. They will probably say that these things are either too antiquated and thus do not relate to modern times or they will say that adolescents are just too rebellious and will not accept the austere, imposing life style and tradition of the Orthodox Church.

I should like to refute the second point by calling your attention to the thousands of adolescents who are running away from home each year. Where are they going? Either they are joining religious groups who first indoctrinate them and then take advantage of their youthful energy or they are being drawn into a life of prostitution - - risking their personal safety.

Some of those who do stay in the home are involved in a merry-go-round life of sex, drugs and crime. With that reality in mind, let us not think that adolescents are too fragile or immature or disinclined to participate in even the most rigorous of Orthodox practices.

In order to refute the premise that Orthodoxy is too antiquated, let us take a brief look at some contemporary literature which addresses the issue of dealing with adolescents:

First is that of Fritz Redl, whose therapeutic remediation for troubled adolescents was based on a structure which involves these three components: routine, rituals, and regulations. Time is important today so I will not elaborate further.

In another Redl technique called the Life-Space Interview, he describes something called the "New Tool Salesmanship."[9] What the concerned adult wants to do is give the adolescent another way of dealing with his conflict and his feelings. A new skill so that he does not continuously find himself in the same predicament over and over again. For instance, fasting can be a new tool for dealing with the body. Although it often seems to the adolescent that his impulses are out of control, fasting lets him know that he/she can be in control despite strong sexual feelings or feelings of anger, aggression or frustration that he may experience. It is not moralizing, sermonizing or judging when an adolescent is offered a tool to help himself. Fasting need not restrict the autonomy which he/she seeks, since he/she will ultimately choose when and what he/she will and will not eat.

Samuel Slavson, in dealing with aggression in boys (and later in girls) proposed for therapeutic use the idea of group balancing.[10] Balance the aggressors with the timid, the volatile with the withdrawn, the interested with the bored, etc., and these personalities will impact on one another and cause positive change. Slavson's implications for church workers is directly related to these dynamics. The different personalities in the community can impact on one another in order to effect positive change and help balance the extremes.

Haim Ginott, without knowing it, supports the need for confession. The sacrament of penance is a healing mystery. The confessor might do what other adults cannot because of their own disappointment or frustration.

In confession the confessor becomes the adolescent's advocate. "Like an attorney, he operates within the law. He does not condone misbehavior or sanction misconduct. A lawyer does not encourage crime. He does not compliment a safe-cracker on his skill or a con man on his cunning. Regardless of the offense, however, he defends the accused. In the most difficult situations he tries

---

[9]Fritz Redl, "The Life Space Interview," American Journal of Orthopsychiatry.

[10]Samuel Slavson, "Differential Methods of Group Therapy in Relation to Age Level," The Nervous Child (New York, New York: Free Press, 1956).

to see the extenuating circumstances and to provide aid and hope."[11] In other works, Ginott describes techniques for congruent communication - - keeping lines of communication open at all times.[12] What could be more Orthodox or modern?

William Glasser, the proponent of reality therapy, while addressing new skills for adolescents, says: "A responsible trainee - - one who comes to work on time, listens to instructions, and helps others - - is more eagerly sought than the trainee with extensive vocational preparation but poor personal characteristics."[13] If we consider the entire process of attending a Divine Service, we see that the adolescent must find out what day of the week and what time the service is to be held, then determine how he/she is going to get there. Before arriving, he/she must be properly attired, have some money to buy a candle, and have the necessary Service book with him/her (if he/she chooses to follow the service). Aside from the spiritual benefits, he/she participates in a process which requires mature behavior but does not add pressure.

There is more that can be said. This presentation is not even an introduction. Let it be sufficient to say that the Orthodox Church is a treasury of knowledge in the sphere of human dynamics. There are models, strategies and interventions for any therapeutic situation. In the meantime, we are seeing that adolescent behavior is becoming more disturbed with each passing decade. Christian families are not immune to these destructive forces, especially as marriages disintegrate at such a high rate.

The Orthodox Church has a tradition of caring for all her members, regardless of their age or situation. If we guide our adolescents back into the fold of the Church, then we can feel assured that they will resolve their conflicts and find identities which will result in effectual and satisfying adulthood.

---

[11] Haim G. Ginott, Between Parent and Teenager (New York, New York: Macmillan and Co., Inc., 1969), p. 64.

[12] Haim G. Ginott, Between Parent and Child (New York, New York: Avon Books, Inc., 1975), p. 19.

[13] William Glasser, Schools Without Failure (New York, New York: Harper and Row, Inc., 1969), p. 251.

II. MEDICINE, PSYCHOLOGY AND RELIGION: NEW DIRECTIONS, NEW INTEGRATIONS

THE UNITY OF BODY, MIND AND SOUL:

A MEDICAL PERSPECTIVE

by Herbert Benson

Good Morning. It is with a great deal of humility that I come to speak at Hellenic College this morning. I am a physician, and yet, as you will see, what I will discuss crosses into areas generally considered to be religion, to a great extent developed under the aegis of the Orthodox Church. I am primarily a translator and what I will be saying is in no way a scientific or mechanistic explanation of prayer but rather a reaffirmation of what religious people have been telling us - - that prayer is good for you. I think such people are correct. Within that context, let me tell you how I, as a physician, became interested in the area of stress, which ultimately led to the definition of the relaxation response, and how that definition led to prayer and, in particular, meditative prayer.

Well over half of us will die in the United States of heart attacks and strokes. Now it is not so disturbing that we are going to die of that disease because, after all, we have to die of something! But what is problematic is that more and more young people are being afflicted with this disease at younger and younger ages. As

---

Dr. Herbert Benson is Associate Professor of Medicine at Harvard Medical School. He is a cardiologist serving as Director of the Division of Behavioral Medicine and the Hypertension Section at Beth Israel Hospital in Brookline, Massachusetts. He is author of the best sellers The Relaxation Response and Body and Mind.

a cardiologist, I became interested in this - - and tried, with many others, to understand what the underlying disease process is so we can do something about it.

The fact that more and more people are dying of this disease was pointed out by several physicians in the 1960's and 1970's in several studies. For example, the late Dr. Samuel Levine, who practiced at the Peter Bent Brigham Hospital noted that the sons of fathers he was treating were developing their heart disease at an average age that was 13 or 14 years younger than their fathers had developed theirs. In other words, the sons were developing heart disease much younger than their fathers had. And then we notice in the hospitals that for the first time, men and women in their 40's and 30's and indeed sometimes in their 20's were coming in with heart attacks and strokes. This was so frequent and so common that the young interns and residents starting their careers thought this to be a matter of course while just five to ten years prior to that to see a heart attack or stroke in a young person would be so rare as to lead to its description in the medical literature.

By far the most common underlying feature in heart attack or stroke is something called atherosclerosis - - or hardening of the arteries. What happens in this process is an artery or aorta, in particular, becomes clogged or blocked; and an artery is the major distributing conduit for the blood. Arteries go to various organs and are carried there from the heart. So if an artery is blocked, the essential nutrients - - oxygen and foodstuffs - - cannot be carried to the organ and the tissues of that organ may die. If this happens in the brain, we are talking about a stroke. If this blockage occurs in one of the heart vessels, the coronary vessels, where what is downstream from the blockage is heart muscle tissue, the tissue may die. This is a "heart attack" - - or a coronary or a myocardial infarction, all meaning the same thing. Should this occur in the kidney, the kidney may become shrunken and diseased.

Alright then, what causes atherosclerosis? There are several major incriminating features. One of them is diet. We have heard a great deal about the amount of cholesterol we eat and the amount of fats in our diet, because these fats are part of the material that ultimately leads to the blockage within the artery. Indeed, we have changed a good part of our national diet because of that. Now we do not eat quite so many fats, specifically, saturated fats; there are many substitutes.

We have been asked to cut down on eggs, butter and other rich foods. The answer cannot, however, be found in diet alone. There are still arguments as to the overall importance, the risk versus benefit, of diet in this process. But there is no question whatsoever that blood pressure is related to atherosclerosis. The higher one's blood pressure, the more rapidly atherosclerosis will develop. The lower one's blood pressure, the more protected one is. Alright, what causes high blood pressure? Here again there are some major problems because over 95% of cases of high blood pressure are due to unknown causes. And for lack of better terms, we call this "essential hypertension;" "hypertension" not meaning being hypertense, but meaning high blood pressure - - and "essential" meaning cause unknown. There are between 23 and perhaps 50 to 60 million adult Americans who suffer from high blood pressure. This is no surprise because when we look at the death rate, we should expect this many people to have high blood pressure; yet, in over 95% of the cases, we do not know the cause of the disease.

A number of years ago, several of us felt that psychological disturbances, that being unable to cope with situations, in short, that stress and its related behavioral adjustments might play an important role in the development of high blood pressure. In fact, this notion has even crept into our speech: "Keep your cool, keep your blood pressure down." But it is extremely difficult to quantify stress; while we can measure blood pressure quite accurately, what would be stressful for one person might not be stressful for another.

More recently, evidence has evolved from a number of different sources; first, from studies of population, epidemiologic studies, where it was shown that under certain circumstances certain people living in the cities tended to have high blood pressure. For example, people living in the cities tended to have higher blood pressure than people living in the country. Take the people from their rural areas, move them into the urban areas, and their blood pressure would increase. At certain times of the year certain groups of people tended to have higher blood pressure. Who for example do you think in this country would have the highest blood pressures as a group around March or April? Accountants and CPA's. When would students have their highest blood pressure? Exam time. Athletes? Before the game. Soldiers? During war, going into battle.

In the Second World War, when the German troops had the city of Leningrad surrounded, people in that city had higher blood pressures when the Germans were there as opposed to after the Germans left. I've often wondered who had the inclination and the time under those circumstances to measure blood pressure, but it was done with a rigid approach. You might remember Texas City, Texas, after the Second World War, in 1948. There were two ships containing ammonia nitrate photosynthesizer which blew up with the force equivalent to several of the bombs dropped on Hiroshima. Windows were damaged within a fifty mile radius with the blast being heard within that range. People within earshot of this developed high blood pressure which lasted about six months and then gradually returned to normal.

More recently, on Three Mile Island, the people living there tended to develop high blood pressure with the threat of nuclear radiation exposure. This kind of thing can be observed in animals as well as people. If you take mice and rats and overcrowd them, they will have higher blood pressure than their own systems can control. Take a mouse, place it in a cage with a hungry cat walking around the cage and that mouse will develop high blood pressure. The Russians did one experiment some of us found disturbing; they put families of baboons, characteristically made up of one male and his harem of females, into a cage. They allowed such a family to become established. Then the removed the original male from the cage, put him in a nearby cage where he could watch, and then replaced him with a new male. Under these somewhat stressful circumstances the original male now watching developed high blood pressure within six weeks and the poor animal died of either a heart attack or a stroke within a year.

We think we understand the mechanism in which such stressful events are translated into high blood pressure. All mammals possess within themselves a response called the emergency response, or the fight or flight response. This resides within an area of the brain called the hypothalamus. And in an area within the hypothalamus, one stimulus leads to a coordinated secretion within the body of adrenaline, and more adrenaline; epinephrine, and more epinephrine; which then leads to a whole host of coordinated changes - - increased heart rate, increased blood pressure, sweating, a three to four hundred percent increase in the amount of blood flow through our muscles, and an increase in our metabolism - - a very important preparedness.

About 60 years ago, Dr. Walter B. Cannon of the Harvard Medical School reasoned that this preparedness was for running or for fighting. Thus the name, the fight or flight response. Under stressful circumstances, we elicit this response. This was most eloquently shown by the Czech physiologist, Dr. Jan Borg. What he did was take healthy medical students, have them lie quietly, and hooked them up to instruments that would measure heart rate, blood pressure, skeletal muscle blood flow and bodily metabolism. Then he told them, "Alright, I want you to do a very simple thing: I'm going to give you a four digit number like 6246. From that

I want you to subtract 17. You're going to get an answer. And from that, subtract 17. And you do that as quickly as possible." The students were also told not to be bothered by a metronome clicking in the background. Click, click, click. Why should you be bothered by your fellow medical students who will give you encouragement? Encouragement that took a form you can well imagine. "You know I can do better than that - - come on let's go." Within two seconds of having to start the substraction, within two seconds of the stimulus, they exhibited the increased heart rate, increased blood pressure, sweating, increased rate of breathing and marked increase in the amount of blood flow through their muscles.

This is the type of situation most of us face daily working under pressure to perform certain tasks. And what has been shown repeatedly is that the elicitation of this response is translated from transient to more or less permanent elevations in blood pressure. Hence the scenario of apparently stressful events, acting through the fight or flight response leading to high blood pressure, later to atherosclerosis and perhaps ultimately to some of the major causes of death we face in the Western World today.

We live in an extremely stressful world under what I believe are the most stressful circumstances man has ever lived. Not that in the past Man did not face death, pestilence and uncertanties, but there was a certain predictability about life. Yes, there were Huns on the horizon or what have you, and one could not predict when a famine would occur, but one lived with and accepted these facts as part of life. In our existence today, we are promised too much; we are almost promised that it is alright to live forever, that it is almost unAmerican to develop a disease.

Our expectations are too high - - but even worse is the unpredictability we have to live with. We do not know from whence stimuli will come, nor do we have standards by which to react to them appropriately. The near assassination of a president, the near assassination of a Pope, rampant violence, the gruesome material in our nightly local news, where the credo of some of the local stations is, "If it bleeds, it leads," where uncertainties come repeatedly . . . take, for example, this Tylenol business. How do you respond to it? You are taking pills. You feel you need the pills and suddenly it is a risk to be taking them. We respond to these events as we are programmed to respond - - with elicitation of the fight or flight response. And ultimately this does us harm, because the response that was once useful, naturally choosing either to run or to fight effectively, no longer serves us because in these situations it is no longer acceptable to run or fight. For example, if you were upset with Tylenol, what would you do about it? Would you hit the person next to you, or start running about the room? Such responses are socially inappropriate, yet our bodies act in such a fashion. Such behavior will breed anxiety and disquiet, inability to get along with others, and a host of symptoms that go along with such disquiet including nausea, vomiting, diarreah, constipation, inability to communicate with others, and the inability to sleep well. These symptoms lead to worsening underlying diseases; if we suffer from something like arthritis, or back pain, or headache, these problems are made worse by stress. What can we do about it?

Fortunately we have within ourselves an opposite response, which is the physiologic opposite to the fight or flight response, and it is this we call the relaxation response. It was first described by a Nobel prize winning Swiss physiologist, Dr. Walter Hess; it was he who found the part of the brain that when stimulated brought forth the fight or flight response that Dr. Cannon described earlier. He found another area within the hypothalamus that when stimulated brought about physiologic changes that were the counterpart, the exact opposite to the fight or flight response. He called this, and I quote, "a protective mechanism against the harmful effects of overstress."

We came upon this in humans about fifteen or so years ago when I was studying in the laboratory of Dr. Barger at the Harvard Medical School. We were working on a model for behaviorally induced high blood pressure through the use of stress. We were able to successfully show that stress could lead to high blood pressure in monkeys. And while these experiments were going on, some young people came to the laboratory and said, esentially, "Why are you fooling around with monkeys? Why don't you study us; we feel we can effectively control our blood pressure. We practice transcendental meditation."

This was 1968, this was the Harvard Medical School; we were having enough trouble convincing people stress could be related to high blood pressure. I told the young people to go away. I really did not want a thing to do with them. Fortunately, they would not leave; they hung around day after day, and insisted that they be studied. Reasoning little would be lost in having a look at whether or not meditation might lead to some physiological changes, we decided to begin our studies of these individuals. And what I shall describe now are some of the physiological changes that occur in this state, but please keep in mind that there is nothing unique about transcendental meditation. As you will see, this state can be achieved in many, many different fashions. But from a historical point of view transcendental meditation was the first description of this state in humans, so let me describe it for you.

About the time we started our experiments Drs. Robert P. Wallis and Archie Wilson started theirs at the University of California. Wallis joined me at Harvard; by pure chance our experimental designs were exactly the same and we were able to collate our data and describe the physiologic changes. The experiments consisted of people coming to the laboratory, having instruments placed on them, intra-arterial needles, catheters and tubes placed in arteries and veins. These instruments measured and collected the amount of gas being expired. Electrodes were placed on their bodies to measure various electrical phenomena, their brain waves being measured by an electroencephelograph. We had the people sit quietly for an entire hour, getting used to the instruments. To begin, for twenty minutes we obtained baseline measurements, the resting measurement. They were then asked to start meditating. They did nothing other than change what they were thinking about; there was no change in their activities, no change in their posture. All they did was start following some meditative instructions. We made other measurements.

Then we asked them to stop meditating and to go back to their regular everyday thoughts. We found rather profound changes. The hallmark of the state is a decrease in the metabolism of the body. There was a 16 to 17 percent decrease from resting, in the amount of oxygen being consumed, that is the amount of fuel being burned by the body. And all that was changed was what the subjects thought about. These changes lasted as long as the subjects followed the meditative instruction. When asked to stop, they returned to baseline or to normal. This was paralleled by decreases in the amount of carbon dioxide being produced, which means that another measure, called respiratory quotient did not change; these people were not hyperventilating (for example, by breathing quickly and holding their breath).

This was a true decrease in the amount of fuel being burned by the body. Also significant was a decrease in the amount of air being moved. In our experiments the subjects' breathing decreased from approximately 13 to 11 breaths per minute. Subsequently, our group as well as others have had the opportunity to measure advanced meditation - - to observe yogis and Tibetan Buddhist monks, whose rate of breathing was down to zero to one breath per minute. Essentially, these individuals stopped breathing for three to four minutes, and then returned to normal without breathing rapidly. There was marked lowering in the amount of fuel being required by the body. And interestingly, the amount of oxygen being carried in the blood to the cells, the amount of "food" to the cells was normal. The cells were getting enough oxygen, they were just using less. Well, we wondered, perhaps we were looking at a state of hibernation. Perhaps man was able to hibernate in a fashion that was previously thought impossible. Another way to look at hibernation, other than looking at the decreased metabolism, is to look at temperature. A hibernating animal will decrease his rectal temperature two to three tenths of a degree. How many of you think bears hibernate? May I have a show of hands? Most of you do. Bears do not hibernate. My reason for asking this is my admiration for two brother physiologists who could determine if bears were sleeping or hibernating in mid-winter. Armed only with rectal thermometers they entered caves where bears were mostly asleep or hibernating, and made their measurements. Indeed, they found out that the bears were sleeping and not hibernating. Continuing their measurements until they woke one of their subjects, who was upset and chased them from the cave, they escaped unharmed and feeling their debt to science had been paid, recorded their results in medical literature. I am fond of that story; I tell it whenever I can.

Under much less hazardous circumstances, we were able to measure rectal temperature in people practicing meditation and found there was no decrease in rectal temperature; therefore, at least in man, this is not a hibernatory state. There were brain wave changes, however; the changes showed a marked slowing and a production of Alpha waves and Theta waves - - very slow waves that have been associated with feelings of peace and tranquility. It is important to recognize that these physiologic changes are distinctly different from those which occur during sleep. For example, in the oxygen consumption decreases that occur within three to five minutes in meditation occur to a lesser degree over four to five hours in sleep, followed by a gradual return to normal.

Brain waves changes are different, as are other bodily metabolic changes. But it did look as if we were having a human counterpart to our tests - - namely, an opposite response to the inborn fight or flight response. If that were the case, it made no sense at all that transcendental meditation would be the only way to bring this about. It would be as if to say there was one way to perspire, or one way to increase one's heartrate, which is silly.

So all we did at that point was look at the four basic steps of transcendental meditation: the first was sit quietly in a comfortable position, the second was close your eyes, the third was have a repetitive word, sound or prayer in your consciousness, and fourth was passively disregard any other thoughts which might come to mind and return to the repetition. Using these four steps as guidelines, we looked to the religious and secular literatures of the world to see whether or not these steps had been described in these texts. What we found, following three to four years of study, was that in virtually every single culture of man, the same exact steps were being practiced.

Let me run through them by way of example: the earliest examples we found were the Ypanishads, the Hindu Scriptures, dating back to the seventh century, B.C., where it was written, "To achieve a union with God, sit quietly by yourself, pay attention to your breathing and on each outbreath say silently to yourself a word from the Scriptures. Should other thoughts come to mind, passively disregard them and come back to the repetitions." The next example we found was within Judaism, dating back to the time of the second temple, which was from the second century, B.C. to the first century, A.D. and within a school of thought called McCaballism. People who were in this school would assume a fetal-like posture - - a sort of squatting - - and rock from heel to toe, on each outbreath repeating over and over the name of the magic seal.

In Christianity, prayers dating back to the time of Christ Himself evolved and were passed on by word of mouth through the monastery, cropping up occasionally and surviving in the Middle Ages; for example, there is a 12th century work - - "The Cloud of Unknowing" - - an anonymous work from England but ultimately being codified on Mount Athos in Greece in the 14th century, where as you know there are Greek Byzantine monasteries. The instructions proscribed twice daily, were sit quietly, pay attention to your breathing, and on each outbreath say silently to yourself, "Lord Jesus Christ, have mercy." Should other thoughts come to mind, passively disregard them and come back to the repetition. Of course, you will recognize this has survived into the modern form that is currently called the Jesus Prayer. At the same time, the 14th century in northern Europe, there was the Jewish catalystic, mystic tradition evolving; and the Rabbi Abulafia, working within that school, wrote, "To achieve the state, sit quietly, pay attention to your breathing, and on each outbreath, say silently to yourself the words, the components, that make up God's name (sounds like Adonai). A similar practice may be found in Islam, where the process is called Bhikr, and a repeated word, a prayer, is called a **wird.**

In Zen Buddhism, people count to ten in magical numbers on each outbreath and then come back to one again over and over, disregarding other thoughts that may come to mind. In Tibetan

Buddhism, people carry prayer beads and throughout the day say the prayer **Om Mani Padmep Hum** over and over - - Hail, jewel of the lotus. Virtually the same thing happens in Shintoism, Taoism, and Confucionism. Only the words are different. In the more primitive, if you will, chauvinistic religions, the same state would be achieved by chanting in time to the stamping of feet or beating of a gong. Here in New England about a hundred years ago there was a school of thought called Nature and Mysticism. Thoreau, Emerson and Alcott belonged to that school close by Concord. They would achieve that state by fixed gazing at light as it shimmered off nearby leaves. Thoreau, on his table at Walden Pond set two books: one was the Hindu Scriptures, the **Bhagavid Gita,** and on many occasions compared himself to a yogi. In England Wordsworth described this beautifully in his poem, "Reflections by Tintern Abbey," where he would achieve this state by fixed gazing at light as it shimmered off a nearby waterfall. Alfred Lord Tennyson, who liked himself a great deal - - used to walk down the street saying his own name over and over - - "Tennyson, Tennyson, Tennyson."

We reasoned that in observing any one of these techniques we might find the same physiologic changes that we found in transcendental meditation. So what we did was go back to the laboratory, bring in some bright Harvard University, Simmons College and Boston College students and give them instructions adapted directly from Zen Buddhism. They were told to sit quietly, close their eyes, pay attention to their breathing and on each outbreath (one, two, three, up to ten, and back to one), passively disregard everyday thoughts when they came to mind.

The experiment was a complete and inexorable failure. What happened was that the bright students lost count, panicked and that was the end of the experiment. We decided to make things simple for them. We asked them to stay with the number one. When we did that, we found exactly the same changes found in transcendental meditation. Next, we brought in people who prayed regularly; not a beseeching prayer asking for something, but: in Catholicism, a Rosary kind of prayer; in Judaism, a devening kind of prayer. We found the same changes. In other words, the prayer, the **sound** used does not matter. If the steps described above are carried out, these physiologic changes will occur. As I stated at the outset, what I am saying here is in no way a scientific or mechanistic explanation of prayer. Rather, it is a reaffirmation of the religious thought of many centuries, that prayer is good for you. As you may now see, such thought is correct.

Our next step was to see whether the regular elicitation of this response had usefulness in the therapy of diseases related to stress - - increased adrenaline, increased neuroadrenaline, increased epinephrine, increased neuroepinephrine; and of course high blood pressure. What we found - - and this has now been verified by at least several designated laboratories - - is that the regular elicitation of the relaxation response, regardless of method, significantly lowers blood pressure. This lowering occurs not only when you are practicing (for example, when you are praying) but carries over into other periods of the day.

Now, if any of you suffer from high blood pressure, you should be taking pills for this, because the drugs lower blood pressure and decrease the risk of atherosclerosis, therefore, decreasing your chances of contracting these other dire diseases. And if you choose to elicit the relaxation response, you should check with your physician first because as you lower your blood pressure your medication might have to be adjusted. Only a physician can appropriately do that. However, if your blood pressure is normal, and you are not taking medications, the side effects of what we are talking about are those of prayer. If prayer is dangerous, this is dangerous.

Prayer has usefulness for patients in many other disease states such as extra heartbeats, or arhythmias. One of my fellow physicians, a Greek Orthodox, was given the number one to repeat in prayer over and over again and his extra heartbeat - - which in this case was quite serious, something called ventricular tachycardia, actually got worse. Observing this, the physician asked, "What is going on?" The patient replied, "Well, this is like voodoo to me. Is there something more compatible that I might use instead of the number one?" So he was wisely given **Kyrie Eleison** and with that his condition markedly improved. The physician used the patient's belief system, and using this, doctor and patient were able to work together.

I will come back to this idea that the word, prayer or phrase you choose should conform to the belief system of the person whom you are teaching. Extra heartbeats, various kinds of arhythmias, most forms of anxiety - - headache, nausea, vomiting, diarreah, insomnia - - the symptoms I mentioned earlier - - inability to get along with others, disquiet . . . these can be cured by sitting quietly once or twice daily and listening to your response. About half the people we worked with who had migraines got significantly better, where the headaches were gone and the others had a significant reduction in their headaches.

It is very useful, even in the therapy of more severe kinds of pain, such as the pain of cancer. It does not make the pain go away, but people are better able to live with the pain. The pain is there, but I recognize there is something in me - - or given to me, if you will - - that is greater than the pain, that allows me to control the pain. And so it is useful in the stress-related disorders that plague our society; while remaining so remarkably simple. It is a natural thing within us; in fact one of the major problems I have in talking about this is the simplicity. It is this very simplicity that gives us problems because in our day and age we are suspect of something that does not cost. We are suspect of something that is natural. People attach gimmicks like machines to this, but it is there simply for the taking to counteract the harmful effects of stress.

As I alluded to earlier, the word, sound, prayer or phrase should be chosen to conform to your belief system, or to the belief system of the person whom you are teaching. The reason for this is that compliance will be better: if you believe in something, it is something you are going to do. Many of my patients at Beth Israel are Roman Catholic. Rather than giving them the number one, I suggest the Jesus Prayer, "Lord Jesus Christ, have mercy." Indeed, these people welcome this. Too many of them say to me, "Thank you doctor, thank you for telling me to pray again. It is something I have wanted to do, but felt funny about; but now that you as a doctor tell me that it is good for me, it is something that I will do." That shows the problems we have in our society.

Then, the compliance of Roman Catholic patients with a prayer they believe in is high. With my Greek Orthodox patients we use **Kyrie Eleison.** With my Jewish patients we use something like Shalom, or echaud meaning one. Protestant patients often choose something from the 23rd Psalm or the Lord's Prayer. For atheistic or agnostic patients, the number one is fine. Others like Eastern techniques, so transcendental meditation is as good as any. What is most important is for the patient to believe in what he is repeating. We have worked hand in glove with many religious organizations of all denominations because meditative prayer is physiologically very healthful. In fact, it is healthful in a way we thought previously was possible only through the use of drugs. What the relaxation response does is actually block - - we learned this recently with Dr. John W. Hoffman a young fellow in our laboratory who recently passed away from leukemia - - norepinephrine or noradrenaline action in a way that some of the most popular drugs now being used in the Western World today do: the beta-blocker syndrome. You do this naturally.

So we have this capacity within us. Here, you teach methods

in your meditative prayer that can bring this about. Bolstered with this physiologic knowledge, I say humbly that perhaps you can use prayer, in addition to its spiritual value, as a valuable tool to promote good health with the regular elicitation of this response.

THE UNITY OF BODY, MIND AND SOUL:

A PASTORAL PSYCHOLOGICAL PERSPECTIVE

by Peter Poulos

It's a great joy for me to be back at Hellenic College today and to participate in this Symposium on Psychology and Religion. The topic for my presentation, "The Unity of Body, Mind and Soul: A Pastoral Psychological Perspective," was not a topic that I chose. It was assigned to me by my good friend, John Chirban. Strangely enough, when I received the brochure with the schedule for the day and saw the topic, I misread it. I read it a number of times for a week as "Body, Mind and Soul: Pastoral Psychological Perspective." I completely missed "The Unity of." Then one day I picked up the schedule, and suddenly I saw this.

I think the reason I missed "The Unity" is because I work in a setting where I do not see the unity of body, mind and soul - - but rather I see the division. I see fragmentation and brokeness. I work in a 550 bed general hospital which is also a teaching hospital with interns and residents. Rather than stay strictly with the topic of "The Unity of Body, Mind and Soul," I would like to describe some of what I see in the hospital - - some of the things that relate to body, some of the things that relate to mind, and some of the things that relate to soul. Then, hopefully, at the end, I

Peter Poulos is a Hospital Chaplain. He serves as Director of Training in Pastoral Care and Clinical Pastoral Education Supervisor at Methodist Hospital, Brooklyn, New York.

will bring these things together and show how they relate to each other.

I hope to describe some emotional or psychological issues that we see in the hospital and the issues that I would call theological issues, noting how these kind of issues relate to each other. I think that the theology of the church definitely has something to say to the modern hospital situation and it is with this that I would want to end my presentation. Let us begin then with a description of what I see in the modern hospital.

I'm not sure how many of you have ever been patients, but it's a strange experience. When you are first admitted they put a name tag on your wrist - - a label that you must wear for identification. This marks your official entrance into that separate world of patient. As a patient, people will come to you dressed in their white uniforms and begin to do things for you and to you. They will give you directions about what you can and cannot do. You give up a lot of your freedom - - you become dependent on other people because you're now a "patient." As a patient you can often feel like a child - - a small child. Tests and procedures are done, often with very large equipment that can at first frighten you. You don't really understand what's going on, even if it's explained. The people around you, the hospital staff, use very technical words - - medical jargon - - that you don't understand. You're in a foreign territory. It's the medical world! Not understanding all the words add to that sense of feeling like a child - - it can add to the confusion, the anxiety.

The anxiety of being a patient though is also partly due to the uncertainty that has now entered your life. Most of us live our life believing that we have some control over it. We do have control over some things in our life. But when illness comes we recognize that we do not have complete control over our life. When tests are being done and we wait for the results, there's a lot of uncertainty. What are they going to find? How much will it change my life? Will I die? What's happening to me? It can be a frightening experience.

Added to the difficulty is the sense of isolation that patients often feel. You're separated from the family - - separated from the people that you work with and from the things you usually do. You can easily feel cut off - - cut off from all the things that make you **you.** One can easily feel that he/she is just a patient - - an object - - a body - - but not a person anymore. I'm not saying that this is always true, but it is often true. We are cut off from the things that make us who we are. From the things that make us the unique persons that we are. From the things that give us some sense of our own identity.

I've heard many patients say - - "I don't feel like myself anymore. I feel like a stranger to myself." That's isolation! That's being cut off! We can also feel cut-off from our own body if there is any significant change in our body image. Changes that occur from a stroke, an amputation, a mastectomy, etc., can make us need to get to know our bodies and body image in a new way. I think the situation that I'm describing raises a lot of concern, theological as well as psychological.

Theological because one of the relationships that often gets changed or challenged by the situation of being a patient, of being ill, is the relationship with God. On the spiritual level there's often a sense of having been abandoned by God - - of being far away from God. Many patients have said, "I can't pray anymore. I pray, but I don't feel like God is here. I can't feel God's nearness." And these are people who could before. In terms of spiritual life, not feeling the presence of God or experiencing Him - - feeling abandoned by God - - is a great threat, a great challenge. On the level of the mind, God also comes in. Because what gets challenged oftentimes is our theology. I've heard many, many patients struggle with their ideas, teachings or beliefs about God, with their theology. Some express an awful lot of anger - -confusion and anger.

We live our life with certain beliefs. For example, many of us were raised with the belief that if we do the right things, if we try to be good Christians, we will be rewarded and that one of the rewards that God will bless us with will be good health and happiness. Suddenly we become ill, or a loved one becomes seriously ill, and our theology is challenged. We wonder, what's going on here? I lived up to my part of the bargain - - where is God? What do I believe? Where is my theology?

Most of us, I think, live in relationship with God in a way in which we want to control God. We work out some kind of a bargain that helps us to control our life. We believe that God, if we do the right things, will also live up to His part of the bargain. And illness is often the time when this is challenged. Such a theology can crumble. The theological dimension of being ill, or of having a loved one who is seriously ill, is that we are faced with our limits. We are faced with the fact that we are human beings - -that we're not God. I've often said to my students (and they laugh at me at the beginning when I say it) that the greatest sin for which I will have to answer to God - - my greatest sin is that deep down in my gut I want to be God. I want to have that power. I want to have that control. I don't want to have limits.

That's something that I struggle with.

I said that my students laugh at me when I say this. That is usually at the beginning of the program. By the time they get to the middle or the end of the program, they realize that they have the same difficulty. They see that they too want to be God - - or want to be able to control God. They see that they too can become frightened and at times angry with their limitations - - the limitations of being human. A big part of what we are dealing with on a daily basis is learning to live with our humanness. Learning to live within the limits and trying to become more comfortable with the fact that we are not all powerful - - that we are not God.

This connects to the other group of people within the hospital that I want to talk about - - this is the staff. Since there are too many staff to talk about, I'll pick one to describe to you briefly; the physician, the doctor. Many physicians struggle with the same thing I've just described: what I would call "wanting to be God." They expect of themselves that they should have all of the answers - - all of the knowledge - - and they have great difficulty when they cannot perform miracles. When they do the best that they could do, the best that anyone could do, and yet the patient dies - - the doctor is confronted with the fact that he or she has limits. In the training of physicians, I don't believe that they are helped to deal with this.

Just the other night an elderly woman died in Intensive Care and the physician who was on the Code procedure when they tried to resuscitate her was having difficulty because she died. This was a woman in her nineties. He was stalling before calling the family doctor and the nurses were getting angry at him. The chaplain who was on duty that night asked, "Is this your first Code where a patient died?" He said, "Yes." He shared that he hadn't thought about what it would be like when this happened. He had never really dealt with it. It's very hard. He and the chaplain talked about this a little, then he went ahead and called the attending doctor. In his head, on an intellectual level, he knew that everything that could have been done for this woman had been done. But, on the feeling level, he felt a sense of failure - - a sense of having been defeated - - and he was struggling with that.

I must tell you I'm glad he was struggling with it because that's a beginning - - at least he was able to talk about it and listen to his own feelings. Many physicians don't. Many physicians have a way of just suppressing their feelings, burying their feelings, and of acting as if they are just a "thinking mind." I make that distinction because the mind is also the seat of feelings, not just of thinking. They function completely on a head level. Just as the patient can become only a body and the person is forgotten, we see the same sin being repeated in the doctor. The doctor becomes just an intellectual being, just a "thinking mind." He or she can be so distant from his or her feelings that at times you cannot sense the person at all. What comes across is a coldness, a lack of sensitivity, a professionalism that is without feeling - - without care. The whole emphasis is on cure. What doesn't get communicated is the care.

There are ways that physicians, and others in the hospital, can create a lot of distance from their own feelings about what is happening. This tends to add to their becoming solely intellectual beings. It adds also to the patient becoming an object, just a body. For example, in the hospital, the staff never refer to a patient as having died; the word is "expired." Very often you will hear a physician say to a family, "I'm sorry to tell you this, but the patient expired." The patient - - not "your husband, or your wife or your daughter." "The patient expired and I have to ask you a question. We want to have permission to do a post-mortem examination" - - which means an autopsy. And all of that is feelingless. "The patient expired" doesn't say anything, and "post-mortem examination" doesn't carry with it the "oomph" or feeling that "autopsy" does. So it's all said in a very distant way.

I wondered whether to share with you an incident that happened recently. I don't want you to think, what kind of hospital is this he works in? I know though from friends working at other hospitals about the many similar things that occur. The incident I wanted to share occurred just last week, a week ago yesterday. It was a very busy afternoon in the Emergency Room and one of the patients died. The medical resident had to go out and tell the husband that his wife had died. He told the wrong man!

You might ask, "How could that happen?" It happened because it was in the Emergency Room - - he didn't know the patient - - the person had just been brought in. The doctor didn't take the time to really find out the name. He was directed to the corridor and was told the husband was waiting there. He told the wrong husband. This happened because of the lack of personal touch. If he had only addressed the man by name, or referred to the patient by name, it would have been clear that it was not this man's wife that he was talking about. But that didn't happen. In this case - - the patient expired. He didn't take the few minutes to find out who is this person, he simply informed a man that his wife's body had died.

I don't want to sound as if I'm bitter against physicians, because I'm not. I really feel for them. I feel for them because they have an awful lot of responsibility. I feel for them because they struggle with much of the same things that I struggle with - - I see a lot of myself in physicians. I want to reach out to them - - help them to be who they are, help them to have their own reactions, their own emotions and to let these come through to people - - not to allow themselves to become just the highly professional machine - - the highly professional thinking but feelingless mind - - that deals with curing bodies.

I mentioned the similarities that I see between myself and physicians; I would say between the clergy and physicians. Clergy struggle with their own limits, much the way physicians do. Clergy get caught up at times in wanting to be God, to be all-powerful, just the way physicians do. People often put clergy on a pedestal and don't expect them to be human. The way the doctor is supposed to have all the answers and be all-wise, the priest or the clergyman is also supposed to be wise and is not felt to be fully human. He should be sinless, perfect.

It's nice to have that illusion, that dream, that someone has all the answers, that someone has reached a level of perfection in life. Many times we put clergy on that pedestal. Clergy live under many of the same struggles and the same pressures that physicians do. Tremendous parallels exist between the two. Both are often very driven - - driven to learn, driven to grow, driven to succeed. Both are separated from other people. Both, by the way, clergy and doctors, often make terrible patients. They don't live very well within limits. It raises an awful lot of anxiety because they are not used to it. They're used to being in a powerful position.

I mentioned earlier how physicians often will use their knowledge in a way that creates some distance from their feelings. One of the things that I see in some clergy and seminary students is this same pattern. They have all the theological answers. Their theology is so solid, but very often a lot of it is out of their head. It is knowledge about God. "Knowledge about" and "experiencing" are not always the same. They can't experience what the patient is experiencing. They don't enter into the patient's experience - - it is foreign to them. They cannot understand what the struggle is. If you have faith, if you have these beliefs, then what are you worried about? What are you anxious about?

This leads to the last part of my presentation which is how theology relates to this human experience - - the experience of brokenness or division between body, mind and soul. The reason I said it leads to this is because I spoke about a struggle and tension. It seems to me that to be a Christian is to be in struggle, to be involved in an "unseen warfare," as one book which talks about spiritual life is so wisely called.

In the early Christian Church there were a number of conflicts or crises which arose, such as Arianism and Nestorianism. These dealt with the person of Jesus Christ. There were questions raised whether He had two natures - - divine and human - - or just one. If He had two natures, was the one stronger than the other? It strikes me that in some ways these questions or issues are still lived out today in relation not to Christ but in regard to what it means to be a human being. We live in a physical world and are physical beings with a body and a mind. But to be human is more than that. We are also spiritual beings. We have the ability to relate with things beyond our own physical limits - - to relate with things even beyond the limited realm of our own personal experience.

This is something that is taught both by theologians and by many psychologists, such as Carl Jung. As human beings made in the image and likeness of God, we can, although being part of the created, relate with our Creator. To be both physical and spiritual beings is to live with some tension between the two. It is to live in a process. As Christians, we live in a world where the Kingdom is here - - but not yet manifest. We await the return of Christ to experience fully the presence of God.

We live in that process where we can experience the Holy Spirit as very close to us one day and so very far away another. To be in process is important both in regard to growth as a person and as a Christian. To be willing to live in the tension, to be willing to live between intimacy/closeness and absence/separation is very much part of our growth as fully human persons and as Christians.

We sin against ourselves, against the way we were created, when we do not recognize and respect the very high calling and high potential we have as human beings. We sin against ourselves when we allow ourselves to become only a body or a mind or a soul, without working toward wholeness and integration. Through the Incarnation of Jesus Christ, we see both our oneness with all of human kind and with all of creation as well as our oneness with Him who made us.

It is very much part of Orthodox theology that life is sacramental, that we are to mark the presence of God in all creation, in all that we do. This is the work of all Christians and particularly of the priest. Our ministry should be incarnational. We are witness to the presence of God, to the presence of Christ in all of life. We are, through our own presence as representatives of the Body of Christ, to represent Christ, to make Christ present again.

At the same time, though, we are to enter into the pain, fear, anxiety and struggle of another person as a "wounded healer," in the way Henri Nouwen, former Professor of Pastoral Theology at Yale Divinity School, describes in his book by that name. When we enter into the brokenness and struggle of another person as wounded healers and truly listen, we recognize that the struggle they are dealing with is not just theirs, but ours. As the psychologist Carl Rogers says in his book <u>On Becoming a Person</u>, "that which is most personal is most universal." We see and hear ourselves in that other person. Through that relationship, a sense of acceptance and community develop, and healing takes place. Not a physical healing necessarily, but a healing that comes with this sense of wholeness and well-being.

I am reminded of the words of Jesus when He said, "He who has seen me has seen the Father" (John 14:9). I believe that when we enter in ministry into the experience of another and truly listen, we can see and hear ourself in that person. Only then can we respond to him/her with genuine sensitivity and care. When this is done in the name of Christ, with an openness to His presence, we also can see and hear Christ. The relationship becomes truly spiritual. The human person is both physical and spiritual . . . and Glory be to God!